Perforator Flaps for Head and Neck Reconstruction

Editor

SUSANA HEREDERO

ORAL AND MAXILLOFACIAL SURGERY CLINICS OF NORTH AMERICA

www.oralmaxsurgery.theclinics.com

Consulting Editor
RUI P. FERNANDES

November 2024 • Volume 36 • Number 4

ELSEVIER

1600 John F. Kennedy Boulevard ● Suite 1800 ● Philadelphia, Pennsylvania, 19103-2899

http://www.oralmaxsurgery.theclinics.com

ORAL AND MAXILLOFACIAL SURGERY CLINICS OF NORTH AMERICA Volume 36, Number 4
November 2024 ISSN 1042-3699, ISBN-13: 978-0-443-31312-7

Editor: John Vassallo; j.vassallo@elsevier.com
Developmental Editor: Anita Chamoli

Oral and Maxillofacial Surgery Clinics of North America (ISSN 1042-3699) is published quarterly by Elsevier Inc., 360 Park Avenue South, New York, NY 10010-1710. Months of issue are February, May, August, and November. Business and Editorial Offices: 1600 John F. Kennedy Blvd., Suite 1800, Philadelphia, PA 19103-2899. Periodicals postage paid at New York, NY and additional mailing offices. Subscription prices are $417.00 per year for US individuals, $100.00 per year for US students/residents, $488.00 per year for Canadian individuals, $100.00 per year for Canadian students/residents, $540.00 per year for international individuals, $235.00 per year for international students/residents. For institutional access pricing please contact Customer Service via the contact information below. To receive student/resident rate, orders must be accompanied by name or affiliated institution, date of term, and the *signature* of program/residency coordinator on institution letterhead. Orders will be billed at individual rate until proof of status is received. Foreign air speed delivery is included in all *Clinics* subscription prices. All prices are subject to change without notice. Orders, claims, and journal inquiries: Please visit our Support Hub page https://service.elsevier.com for assistance.

Reprints. For copies of 100 or more, of articles in this publication, please contact the Commercial Reprints Department, Elsevier Inc., 360 Park Avenue South, New York, NY 10010-1710. Tel.: 212-633-3874; Fax: 212-633-3820; Email: reprints@elsevier.com.

Oral and Maxillofacial Surgery Clinics of North America is covered in *MEDLINE/PubMed* (*Index Medicus*), *Science Citation Index Expanded (SciSearch®)*, *Journal Citation Reports/Science Edition*, and *Current Contents®/Clinical Medicine*.

Contributors

CONSULTING EDITOR

RUI P. FERNANDES, MD, DMD, FACS, FRCS(Ed)
Clinical Professor and Chief, Division of Head and Neck Surgery, Program Director, Head and Neck Oncologic Surgery and Microvascular Reconstruction Fellowship,
Departments of Oral and Maxillofacial Surgery, Neurosurgery, and Orthopaedic Surgery and Rehabilitation, University of Florida Health Science Center, University of Florida College of Medicine, Jacksonville, Florida, USA

EDITOR

SUSANA HEREDERO, MD, PhD, FEBOMFS
Consultant Maxillofacial Surgeon, Department of Maxillofacial Surgery, Hospital Universitario
Reina Sofía, Unidad de Cirugía Reconstructiva Avanzada, Hospital Cruz Roja, Paseo de la Victoria s/n, Córdoba, Spain

AUTHORS

ANDREW ATIA, MD
Fellow, Department of Plastic Surgery, The University of Texas MD Anderson Cancer Center, Houston, Texas, USA

ALESSANDRO BIANCHI, MD
Plastic Surgeon, UOSD Chirurgia Plastica, Dipartimento Salute Donna, Bimbo e Sanità Pubblica, Università Cattolica del "Sacro Cuore" – Fondazione Policlinico Universitario "Agostino Gemelli" IRCSS, Rome, Italy

BENIAMINO BRUNETTI, MD, PhD
Surgeon, Plastic, Reconstructive and Aesthetic Surgery Department, Campus Bio-Medico University, Rome, Italy

WEI F. CHEN, MD, FACS
Professor and Co Director of Center for Lymphedema Research and Reconstruction, Department of Plastic and Reconstructive Surgery, Cleveland Clinic, Cleveland, Ohio, USA

HARVEY CHIM, MD, FACS
Professor, Plastic Surgery and Neurosurgery, Division of Plastic and Reconstructive Surgery, Department of Surgery, University of Florida, Gainesville, Florida, USA

JONG WOO CHOI, MD, PhD, MMM
Professor, Department of Plastic and Reconstructive Surgery, University of Ulsan College of Medicine, Asan Medical Center, Seoul, Korea

LINDA CHOW, MD, FRCSC
Head and Neck Surgical Oncology and Microvascular Surgery Fellow, Department of Otolaryngology–Head and Neck Surgery, University of Florida, Gainesville, Florida, USA

PETER DZIEGIELEWSKI, MD, FRCSC, FACS
Kenneth W. Grader Professor in Head and Neck Surgery, Chief of Head and Neck Oncologic and Microvascular Reconstructive Surgery, Fellowship Director, Advanced Head and Neck Oncologic Surgery, University of Florida, Gainesville, Florida, USA

RAMI ELMORSI, MD
Postdoctoral Fellow, Department of Plastic Surgery, The University of Texas MD Anderson Cancer Center, Houston, Texas, USA

MARIA ISABEL FALGUERA, MD, FEBOMFS
Consultant Maxillofacial Surgeon, Unidad de Cirugía Reconstructiva Avanzada, Hospital Cruz Roja, Paseo de la Victoria s/n, Córdoba, Spain

VICENÇ GÓMEZ, MD
Consultant Maxillofacial Surgeon, Department of Maxillofacial Surgery, Hospital Universitario Vall d'Hebron, Barcelona, Spain

LAURENT GANRY, MD, MSc, FEBOMFS
Department of Oral and Maxillofacial Surgery, Donald and Barbara Zucker School of Medicine, Long Island Jewish Medical Center, New Hyde Park, New York, USA

MIGUEL ANGEL GAXIOLA-GARCIA, MD
Attending Plastic Surgeon, Hospital Infantil de México "Federico Gómez" (Mexico's Children's Hospital), Mexico City, Mexico

STEFANO GENTILESCHI, MD
Associate Professor in Plastic Surgery, Chief, UOSD Chirurgia Plastica, Dipartimento Salute Donna, Bimbo e Sanità Pubblica, Università Cattolica del "Sacro Cuore" – Fondazione Policlinico Universitario "Agostino Gemelli" IRCSS, Rome, Italy

AKITATSU HAYASHI, MD
Plastic Surgeon, Department of Breast Center, Kameda Medical Center, Kamogawa, Chiba, Japan

SUSANA HEREDERO, MD, PhD, FEBOMFS
Consultant Maxillofacial Surgeon, Department of Maxillofacial Surgery, Hospital Universitario Reina Sofía, Unidad de Cirugía Reconstructiva Avanzada, Hospital Cruz Roja, Paseo de la Victoria s/n, Córdoba, Spain

TAREK ISMAIL, MD PD
Senior Physician, Division of Plastic, Reconstructive, Aesthetic and Hand Surgery, Department of Surgery, University Hospital of Basel, Basel, Switzerland

CYRUS KERAWALA, FDSRCS, FRCS (OMFS), RCPathME
Professor, Consultant Maxillofacial, Head and Neck Surgeon, Head and Neck Unit, The Royal Marsden NHS Foundation Trust, London, United Kingdom

YOUNG CHUL KIM, MD
Assistant Professor, Department of Plastic and Reconstructive Surgery, University of Ulsan College of Medicine, Asan Medical Center, Seoul, Korea

SONIA KUKREJA-PANDEY, MD
Lymphatic Supermicrosurgery Fellow, Department of Plastic Surgery, Cleveland Clinic, Cleveland, Ohio, USA

RENE D. LARGO, MD
Associate Professor, Department of Plastic Surgery, The University of Texas MD Anderson Cancer Center, Houston, Texas, USA

Z-HYE LEE, MD
Assistant Professor, Department of Plastic Surgery, The University of Texas MD Anderson Cancer Center, Houston, Texas, USA

MATTEO MERONI, MD
Department of Health Sciences and Medicine, University of Lucerne, Lucerne, Switzerland; Plastic Surgery Resident, Zentrum für Plastische Chirurgie, Pyramid Clinic, Klinik Pyramide am See, Zürich, Switzerland

ANTONIO MESCHINO, MSc
Faculty of Medicine of Vilnius University, Vilnius, Lithuania; Faculty, Dipartimento di Chirurgia, Ospedale Regionale di Locarno, Locarno, Switzerland

NISHAN MOHEEPUTH, MD
Specialist Plastic Surgeon, Med Esthetique, Petit Raffray, Mauritius

JINGYA JANE PU, BDS, MDS
Clinical Assistant Professor, Division of Oral and Maxillofacial Surgery, Faculty of Dentistry, The University of Hong Kong, Prince Philip Dental Hospital, Sai Ying Pun, Hong Kong

GUNESH P. RAJAN, MD, DM, FRACS
Clinical Professor, Department of Otolaryngology, Head and Neck Surgery, Luzerner Kantonsspital, Lucerne, Switzerland; Otolaryngology, Head and Neck Surgery, Medical School, University of Western Australia, Perth, Australia

FRANCESCO M.G. RIVA, MD, FRCS
Head and Neck/Reconstructive Associate Specialist, Head and Neck Unit, The Royal Marsden NHS Foundation Trust, London, United Kingdom

ANDRES RODRIGUEZ-LORENZO, MD, PhD
Head of Department, Associate Professor, Department of Plastic and Maxillofacial

Surgery, Uppsala University, Consultant, Department of Surgical Sciences, Uppsala University Hospital, Uppsala, Sweden

MARZIA SALGARELLO, MD
Associate Professor in Plastic Surgery, UOSD Chirurgia Plastica, Dipartimento Salute Donna, Bimbo e Sanità Pubblica, Università Cattolica del "Sacro Cuore" – Fondazione Policlinico Universitario "Agostino Gemelli" IRCSS, Rome, Italy

ALBA SANJUAN-SANJUAN, MD, PhD, FEBOMFS
Consultant Maxillofacial Surgeon, Oral and Maxillofacial Surgery, Charleston Area Medical Center, Charleston, West Virginia, USA

MARIO F. SCAGLIONI, MD
Professor, Department of Health Sciences and Medicine, University of Lucerne, Lucerne, Switzerland; Co-Chief, Zentrum für Plastische Chirurgie, Pyramid Clinic, Klinik Pyramide am See, Zürich, Switzerland

YU-XIONG SU, MD, PhD
Clinical Professor, Division of Oral and Maxillofacial Surgery, Faculty of Dentistry, The University of Hong Kong, Prince Philip Dental Hospital, Sai Ying Pun, Hong Kong

JEREMY MINGFA SUN, MBBS, MRCS, MMeD, FAMS
Consultant, Plastic, Reconstructive and Aesthetic Surgery Service, Department of Surgery, Changi General Hospital, Singapore, Singapore

LUÍS VIEIRA, MD, MSc
Assistant, Department of Plastic, Reconstructive and Aesthetic Surgery, Central Lisbon University Hospital, Lisbon, Portugal

GIUSEPPE VISCONTI, MD, PhD
Plastic Surgeon, UOSD Chirurgia Plastica, Dipartimento Salute Donna, Bimbo e Sanità Pubblica, Università Cattolica del "Sacro Cuore" – Fondazione Policlinico Universitario "Agostino Gemelli" IRCSS, Rome, Italy

HAO-I. WEI, MD
Plastic Surgery Resident, Department of Plastic Surgery, Chang Gung Memorial Hospital, Taipei, Taiwan

FU-CHAN WEI, MD, FACS
Distinguished Chair Professor, Department of Plastic Surgery, Chang Gung Memorial Hospital, Chang Gung University Medical College, Taoyuan, Taiwan

LUCCIE M. WO, MD, MS
Microsurgery Fellow, Department of Plastic Surgery, Chang Gung Memorial Hospital, Masters in Reconstructive Microsurgery Candidate, Chang Gung University, Taoyuan City, Taiwan; Assistant Professor, Division of Plastic and Reconstructive Surgery, Department of Surgery, Yale School of Medicine, New Haven, Connecticut, USA

TAKUMI YAMAMOTO, MD, PhD
Head, Department of Plastic and Reconstructive Surgery, Center Hospital of National Center for Global Health and Medicine, Shinjuku-ku, Tokyo, Japan

PEIRONG YU, MD, MS, FACS
Professor and Chair ad Interim, Department of Plastic Surgery, The University of Texas MD Anderson Cancer Center, Houston, Texas, USA

Contents

The Past, Present, and Future of Perforator Flaps in Head and Neck Surgery 425

Luccie M. Wo, Hao-I. Wei, and Fu-Chan Wei

A perforator is a vessel that travels through muscle and perfuses the skin. Perforator flaps require intramuscular dissection and can be used as pedicled or free flap. With improved understanding of microvasculature, they can be tailored to have multiple skin paddles, multiple components, or shaped to conform to any defect. Reliable perforator flap-based reconstruction is a meticulous microvascular technique, ultimately allowing the surgeon to harvest any flap in a freestyle fashion and transplant to any recipient vessel. New technologies improve the safety and reproducibility of this type of reconstruction.

Functional Perspectives in Tongue Reconstruction Based on Perforator Free Flap 435

Jong Woo Choi and Young Chul Kim

This article explores advancements in functional tongue reconstruction after cancer ablation, focusing on the importance of flap selection, positioning, and volume adjustment to restore speech and swallowing function. It highlights advancements such as the perforator flap concept for customized reconstructions and the transition to dynamic techniques with motor-innervated free flaps, aiming to accurately replicate the tongue's inherent functions. The effectiveness of dynamic techniques in improving swallowing efficiency and speech clarity underscores their significant potential in enhancing postoperative rehabilitation, representing a significant progress in the realm of functional tongue reconstruction.

The Anterolateral Thigh Flap in Head and Neck Reconstruction 451

Jingya Jane Pu, Andrew Atia, Peirong Yu, and Yu-Xiong Su

The anterolateral thigh (ALT) free flap has become a workhorse for head and neck reconstruction. This paper offers a thorough introduction to the ALT flap, covering its anatomy, surgical technique, adaptable designs, and use in a range of clinical settings along with case studies. With its long vascular pedicle and tissue versatility, the ALT flap is well-suited for matching varied defects. Still, understanding possible anatomic variances and managing complications are critical to its success. With this paper as a comprehensive guidance, surgeons can apply the ALT flap for difficult head and neck reconstructions and achieve the best possible results.

The Role of Deep Inferior Epigastric Perforator and Thoracodorsal Artery Perforator Flaps in Head and Neck Reconstruction 463

Luís Vieira and Andres Rodriguez-Lorenzo

Head and neck reconstruction has evolved to a more accurate replacement of the missing tissues for aesthetic and functional benefits, besides a concern with the morbidity caused in the donor site. This has led us to the use of perforator flaps. Deep inferior epigastric perforator flap allows the harvest of a large well-vascularized skin paddle with adequate bulk for large and voluminous defects reconstruction. Its main uses described in the literature are: tongue reconstruction, orbitomaxillary reconstruction, and scalp reconstruction. Thoracodorsal artery perforator flap is derived from the subscapular system and allows the harvest of a large array of chimeric flaps.

Reconstructive surgeons navigate a plethora of options when choosing a soft-tissue flap donor site for head and neck reconstruction, each with its distinct pros and cons. This review delves into the profunda artery perforator flap and provides expert recommendations for its use in head and neck reconstruction.

Head and neck defects present a unique challenge in reconstructive surgery due to the complex anatomy of this area. Different defects often require a variety of reconstructive techniques. The superficial circumflex iliac artery perforator (SCIP) flap is particularly notable for its versatility in this context. It provides a thin, pliable skin island that can be integrated with bone, muscle, fascia, and other structures. Additionally, the morbidity associated with the donor site of the SCIP flap is generally low and well tolerated. This article offers a comprehensive overview of the evolution of this technique.

This article illustrates the use of locoregional perforator and pedicled flaps from the 2 main vascular systems of the head and neck area. The 2 authors combine their experiences and research findings to highlight clinical scenarios for these useful refined reconstructions and discuss their pros and cons.

Microsurgeons have today the freedom of the "chosen flap," as opposed to the "flap of choice," but the preoperative knowledge of the microanatomy of each patient is mandatory. The need for preoperative evaluation of the perforators, not only in terms of position, but also for dimensions, flow, and relationship with the surrounding structures became essential and allows more personalized reconstruction, less invasiveness, more safety and finally increase microsurgeon creativity.

Preoperative computed tomography angiography (CTA) for perforator free flaps is accurate, precise, and reliable in mapping perforator anatomy that can be used in the intraoperative domain. CTA holds important clinical value as a tool in surgical decision making and surgical innovation, enabling reconstructive surgeons to tailor complex flap designs for extensive defects. Integration into existing infrastructure for virtual surgical planning is feasible, and future efforts to characterize the association of preoperative CTA with postoperative outcomes and cost-analyses for perforator flaps are warranted.

The authors aim to provide a comprehensive overview of the advancements in head and neck reconstructive surgery using thinned perforator flaps. The article categorizes these flaps based on thickness and discusses the importance of standardized terminology. Critical aspects like flap vascularity, pre-operative planning, and imaging technologies for perforator mapping are examined with practical considerations. The article then delves into various thinning techniques and their applications in head and neck reconstructions, highlighting challenges and concerns. In conclusion, significant progress in reconstructive surgery using thinned perforator flaps has brought advancements in improving surgical precision and patient outcomes in head and neck reconstructions.

 Video content accompanies this article at http://www.oralmaxsurgery.theclinics.com.

The integration of imaging technologies such as computed tomography angiography and color Doppler ultrasonography are transforming soft tissue free flap reconstruction. The search for thinner and more refined flaps has expanded indications for flaps harvested from donor sites that were not commonly used in head and neck reconstruction. This article explores how these tools and techniques facilitate precise flap selection, thickness, and design customization based on detailed patient preoperative perforator anatomy and vascular configuration mapping. Optimizing outcomes with tailored flap designs improves surgical accuracy and patient-specific results in soft tissue reconstruction.

Head and neck cancer (HNC) is the sixth most common cancer across the world. Despite a general reduction in tobacco consumption and therefore reduction in risk exposure there has been an increasing incidence of oropharyngeal squamous cell carcinoma. Progress made in the past decades in free tissue transfer reconstruction and robotic surgery have merged into transoral robotic reconstruction with free perforator flaps for head and neck. We reviewed and discussed indications and contraindications for this type of procedure, as well as potential limits refinements.

In this study, the authors shed light on the underappreciated realm of head and neck lymphedema (HNL) amid the backdrop of significant advancements in extremity lymphedema management. Despite its prevalence and impact, HNL has long been overlooked, attributed to its subtle symptom presentation and lack of awareness among primary care providers. The study delves into the unique challenges associated with diagnosing and treating HNL, emphasizing the predominance of internal swelling over external manifestations. The authors advocate for the refinement and standardization of outcome measures and the integration of innovative techniques such as indocyanine green lymphography and patient-reported outcomes.

ORAL AND MAXILLOFACIAL SURGERY CLINICS OF NORTH AMERICA

SERIES OF RELATED INTEREST

Atlas of the Oral and Maxillofacial Surgery Clinics
www.oralmaxsurgeryatlas.theclinics.com

Dental Clinics
www.dental.theclinics.com

THE CLINICS ARE NOW AVAILABLE ONLINE!
Access your subscription at:
www.theclinics.com

Preface

Transformative Techniques in Microsurgical Soft Tissue Head and Neck Reconstruction: Commitment and Passion

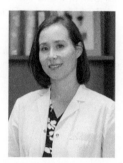

Susana Heredero, MD, PhD, FEBOMFS
Editor

This issue of *Oral and Maxillofacial Surgery Clinics of North America* focuses on the intricate and evolving field of perforator flaps in head and neck (H&N) reconstruction. H&N reconstruction is a highly demanding specialization, requiring deep commitment and inexhaustible dedication, but it can dramatically enhance the quality of life for our patients. Despite these demands, the unwavering commitment to advancing patient care remains paramount. I would like to express my sincere appreciation to all the authors who have contributed to this issue with their time and knowledge, sharing their expertise, creative insight, and passion for microsurgical reconstruction.

The content includes a collection of articles, starting with a comprehensive overview of the past, present, and future directions on using perforator flaps in H&N. Then, we delve into the details and application of the workhorse and other innovative perforator free flaps, which have expanded our armamentarium and resources to achieve the best functional and aesthetic results. This journey of evolution in H&N reconstructive microsurgery has also been closely related to technological developments in recent years. Advancements in imaging techniques have not only significantly enhanced the precision and success of perforator flap harvesting but also allowed us to pursue more sophisticated and safer reconstructions. In addition, robotic-assisted surgery has facilitated flap inset and reduced the morbidity of surgical access in certain anatomical reconstruction sites. Finally, lymphedema surgery is one of the future developing fields in reconstructive H&N microsurgery. H&N lymphedema is a condition that is often overlooked or misdiagnosed. Moreover, the implication

Oral Maxillofacial Surg Clin N Am 36 (2024) xi–xii
https://doi.org/10.1016/j.coms.2024.07.010
1042-3699/24/© 2024 Published by Elsevier Inc.

of brain lymphatics in cognitive dysfunction is a new, promising research field.

I want to thank the editorial team of *Oral and Maxillofacial Surgery Clinics of North America* for their trust and support throughout the creation of this project. I am grateful to Dr Rui Fernandes for being an inspiring mentor and allowing me to contribute to this journal. I would also like to thank John Vassallo and Anita Chamoli for their guidance, patience, perseverance, and invaluable work. It has been a great pleasure working with such dedicated professionals.

I hope this issue will inspire you to improve patient care, explore your creative ideas, and continue working in the exciting world of H&N reconstructive microsurgery.

DISCLOSURES

The author has no financial interest in the products, devices, or drugs mentioned in this article. The study was not financially supported by any grants.

Susana Heredero, MD, PhD, FEBOMFS
Unidad de Cirugía Reconstructiva Avanzada
del Hospital Cruz Roja de
Córdoba, Spain

Maxillofacial Surgery Department
Hospital Universitario Reina Sofía
Avd Menéndez Pidal s/n
Córdoba 14004, Spain

E-mail address:
susana_heredero@yahoo.es

The Past, Present, and Future of Perforator Flaps in Head and Neck Surgery

Luccie M. Wo, MD, MS[a,b], Hao-I. Wei, MD[c,1], Fu-Chan Wei, MD[d,*]

KEYWORDS

• Perforator flap • Hand neck reconstruction • ALT flap

KEY POINTS

• Reconstruction of composite defects of the head and neck frequently require microsurgical techniques with the anterior lateral thigh free flap being one of the most used perforator flaps for soft tissue reconstruction.
• A perforator flap is a skin flap that is perfused by a vessel that has an intramuscular course. Mastery of the intramuscular dissection enables the surgeon to elevate almost any soft tissue flap.
• Better understanding of microsurgical anatomy and new technology have been developed to improve the safety and predictability of free flap reconstruction.

INTRODUCTION

Since the first description of perforator flaps in 1989, they have gradually become routinely used flaps for head and neck reconstruction. As our understanding of perforators and angiosomes evolved, we have further pushed the boundaries of these flaps: expanding their indication, creating customized chimerization, and better tailoring each flap to the demands of reconstruction. In this article, the authors will describe the history of its evolution, the current applications, and explore new possible innovations in the future.

HISTORY OF PERFORATOR FLAPS

Coining of the Term "Perforator Flap" and What's a True "Perforator Flap"

With the progression of microscopic techniques, the idea of the free flap was born where surgeons can harvest tissue with a vessel pedicle and transplant it to a new site by performing a microvascular anastomosis to existing vessels at the recipient site. Initially, this was only performed for soft tissue with named vessels, such as muscle and omentum. However, as reconstructive surgeons became more sophisticated with microsurgical techniques, smaller vessels became contenders for microvascular transplantation. The concept and technique of the "pedicled skin flap" evolved from the random pattern flap when Milton[1] discovered that flap survival was dependent on the inclusion of a pedicled blood vessel. Basically, the pedicle to the skin flap in the past used to be a distal branch of a source vessel (direct vessel) or have its course between 2 muscles (septocutaneous vessel). In 1987, Taylor and Palmer organized our understanding of skin vessels territories into angiosomes.[2] Taylor's research generated a detailed anatomic description of the skin vasculature and identified 374 vessels to the skin with diameters greater than 0.5 mm, which are all feasible candidate for microvascular anastomosis. Thus,

[a] Department of Plastic Surgery, Chang Gung Memorial Hospital, Chang Gung University; [b] Division of Plastic and Reconstructive Surgery, Department of Surgery, Yale School of Medicine, 800 Howard Avenue, 4th Floor, New Haven, CT 06519, USA; [c] Department of Plastic Surgery, Chang Gung Memorial Hospital; [d] Department of Plastic Surgery, Chang Gung Memorial Hospital, Chang Gung University Medical College, 5, Fu-Hsing Street, Guishan, Taoyuan 333, Taiwan
[1] Present address: No. 428, Houzhuang Road, Touliu City, Yunlin, Taiwan.
* Corresponding author.
E-mail address: fuchanwei@gmail.com

Oral Maxillofacial Surg Clin N Am 36 (2024) 425–433
https://doi.org/10.1016/j.coms.2024.07.003
1042-3699/24/© 2024 Elsevier Inc. All rights are reserved, including those for text and data mining, AI training, and similar technologies.

each of these is a potential donor site for a skin flap.

The latest version of the free flap is the "perforator flap." The terminology was first coined by Koshima and Soeda in 1989 in a landmark paper that described the inferior epigastric artery skin flap without inclusion of the rectus abdominis muscle.[3] The main advantage of the perforator flap over more traditional musculocutaneous flap is the reduced donor site morbidity leading to faster postoperative recovery. However, perforator flaps do require dissection in the muscle to expose the pedicle, in some cases a small cuff of muscle is also taken to protect the pedicle vessel. Elevation of a perforator flap does require meticulous intramuscular dissection, often done with loupe or microscope magnification.

Nomenclature of Perforators Flaps and Controversies

As our understanding of skin flaps expanded, additional categorization of vessels that perfuse the skin were recognized. In 1986, Nakajima already described 6 different subtypes of fasciocutaneous flaps based on the characteristics of the vessel perfusing the skin. The 6 subtypes include the direct cutaneous flap (type I), the direct septocutaneous flap (type II), the perforating cutaneous branch of muscle vessel flap (type III), direct cutaneous branch of muscle vessel flap (type IV), septocutaneous perforator flap (type V), and musculocutaneous perforator (type VI).[4] Although from the surgical dissection technique point of view, differentiating type III, IV, and V from type VI is unnecessary.

The term perforator has been used to describe any vessel that perfuses the skin: this is incorrect. In its purest form, a perforator is a blood vessel that originates from a named source vessel, travels through a named muscle, and extends to perfuse the skin. Thus, the authors advocate that a perforator flap should only refer to pure skin flaps perfused by a vessel that requires intramuscular dissection. Flaps based on direct cutaneous vessels or septal vessels do not require any intramuscular dissection for elevation. Instead, these flaps are named direct vessel-based or septal vessel-based flap. In 2003, the Gent Consensus[5] sought to include vessels other than myocutaneous ones as various types of perforator flaps which the senior author (FCW) considers as redundant and even leading to confusion in communications. This difference is important as the muscle dissection for a musculocutaneous perforator flap is significantly more technically challenging and time consuming than a septocutaneous or direct vessel-based flap. The true perforator flaps have

been named after tits surface anatomy location, the muscle through which the pedicle transverses, or its source vessel. There is still no consensus yet on the naming system for perforator flaps.

CURRENT DEVELOPMENTS OF PERFORATOR FLAPS IN HEAD AND NECK RECONSTRUCTION
Work-Horse Flap for Head and Neck Reconstruction

Microsurgical free flap reconstruction has gradually become the standard-of-care for reconstruction since its first description in 1980s. While many flaps have been described, currently, the 3 main workhorse flaps for soft tissue and bone reconstruction are the anterolateral thigh (ALT) flap, radial forearm flap, and fibula flap. These flaps are favored as free flaps because they generally have a large and long pedicle with consistent anatomy, potential to include a diverse tissue type on a single pedicle, easy and straightforward dissection, acceptable donor site morbidity, and allow for 2-team approach.

In this context, the ALT flap is the model perforator flap, particularly for soft tissue reconstruction. Other perforator flaps from the lower extremity for head and neck reconstruction include the profunda artery perforator (PAP) flap and the anterior medial thigh (AMT) flap. The ALT flap is one of the most versatile flaps available. It can be harvested with a large skin paddle which can then be tailored and folded for a multitude of applications. The ALT can be raised in either suprafascial or subfascial plane, and even after elevation it can be thinned during the index surgery. The ALT flap may also be designed as a chimeric flap with inclusion of the vastus lateralis muscle, which may be necessary for reconstructing extensive composite defects. Thus, the ALT flap is one of the most used workhorse flaps for soft tissue head and neck reconstruction.

Anterolateral Thigh Flap

The ALT flap is based on the descending branch of the lateral circumflex femoral artery and it was first described as a flap with septocutaneous vessels by Song in 1984.[6] However, septocutaneous vessels feeding the ALT flap can only be found in 13% to 18% of cases.[7] The more common anatomic variation is musculocutaneus perforators, usually 1 to 3 perforators (**Fig. 1**) approximately 1 mm in diameter.[7] The ALT flap can be harvested as a perforator-based skin flap, a myocutaneous flap, a muscle flap, or a chimeric flap (**Fig. 2**). It can also be customized to be a sensate flap, flow through flap, and functional muscle flap.

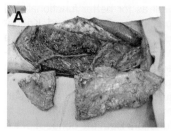
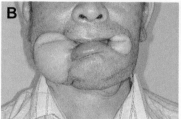
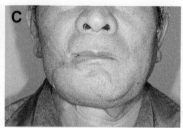

Fig. 1. (A) Two anterolateral thigh (ALT) flaps elevated from the same donor site. (B) Appearance 1 month after bilateral mouth angles cancer excision and ALT flap reconstruction. (C) Appearance after bilateral oral commissuroplasty.

Depending on the number and characteristics of the perforators included in the flap, enormous skin paddle can be harvested. Some of the largest described in literature are 400 to 720 cm².[8] The senior author (FCW) usually harvests an 8 × 22 cm skin paddle, which is large enough to reconstruct approximately 95% of soft tissue defects in the head and neck. During the 2-team approach, the flap harvest often commences before the malignancy resection is complete; therefore, it is advantageous to harvest a large soft tissue flap that can then be further tailored during inset. Furthermore, large flaps are often needed to obliterate dead space: that is, the maxilla sinus following a maxillectomy or the floor of mouth after a tongue resection. In such scenarios, the ALT flap can be de-epithelialized and folded to obliterate dead space and avoid the shrunken appearance. Furthermore, larger flaps also mitigate the shrinkage effects of postoperative radiation.

It is important to balance the benefits of harvesting a large ALT flap with morbidity to the donor site. If a larger skin paddle is harvested, the donor site will require a skin graft for closure. Skin grafting at the donor site can result in limitation of range of motion at the hip and knee due to adhesions between the skin graft and underlying tissue.[9] If skin grafting is to be avoided, the ALT flap should not be wider than 8 cm in adults.

Harvesting the ALT flap starts with identifying the anterior superior iliac spine and the superior lateral border of the patella. A line can be drawn between these 2 landmarks and the main cutaneous vessels are centered at the halfway point. Doppler ultrasound can be used to detect the vessels preoperatively and a flap can be designed around the location of the skin vessels (**Fig. 3**). The most described approach to elevation starts with an exploratory medial incision above the rectus femoris muscle. By not committing to a posterior incision at the same time, the surgeon can modify the skin pattern design after having visualized and dissected the selected perforator(s). Dissection can be taken down to the level of the fascia and the perforators can be identified in the suprafascial or subfascial plane. In some cases, a sizable septocutaneous vessel feeding the skin is identified; selecting this vessel can reduce both donor site morbidity and operative time as no intramuscular dissection is needed. In the majority of cases, the intramuscular course of the perforator is approximately 6 to 10 cm.[7] The cutaneous perforator is usually traced back to the descending branch of the lateral circumflex artery, which lies between the vastus lateralis and rectus femoris muscle. If a sensate flap is needed, the lateral femoral cutaneous nerve innervating the flap can be included.

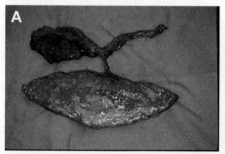
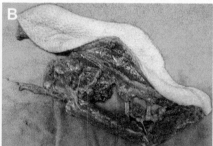

Fig. 2. Chimeric flaps contain 2 or more different components, each tissue component must have a defined pedicle with an independent blood supply, and the tissue components and their pedicles are naturally linked. (A) Chimeric flap from the lateral circumflex femoral system with inclusion of skin and vastus lateralis muscle. (B) Chimeric flap from the peroneal system with inclusion of skin, fibula bone, and soleus muscle.

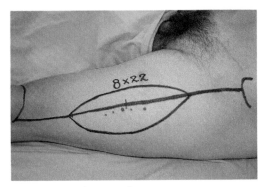

Fig. 3. Design of an ALT flap.

Infrequently, no sizable perforators can be found (or if the ALT perforators are damaged), the surgeon can convert to a tensor fascia lata flap or the AMT flap.[10] The tensor fascia lata flap receives blood supply from the transverse branch of the lateral circumflex femoral artery. The main blood supply to the AMT flap is the rectus femoris branch, which comes from the descending lateral circumflex femoral artery. In fact, anatomic studies demonstrated that patients with 1 or fewer ALT perforator had a 4-fold increased chance of an AMT perforator.[10]

With mastery of the ALT flap and perforator flap intramuscular dissection techniques, the reconstructive surgeon can harvest almost all kinds of soft tissue flaps for head and neck reconstruction. On average, the human body has 374 vessels with diameter greater than 0.5 mm, which in theory translates to 374 potential flaps.[2] It is impossible to learn and perform all these flaps in a surgical training. Instead, mastery of the workhorse flaps should focus on how to select a proper flap, how to select a sizable perforator, how to skillfully perform an intramuscular dissection, and how to reliably perform microsurgical anastomosis. Certain tools such as Doppler, ultrasound, and CT angiography can help with perforator mapping, aiding the surgeon in preoperative flap design. Once this skill set is mastered, a reconstructive surgeon will have the ability to elevate almost any flap.

Reconstructive Elevator

The reconstructive ladder can be traced back to before the ancient Egyptians.[11] The principle of a reconstructive ladder is to use the simplest means to obtain an acceptable wound coverage. One should go up to a higher rung, or more complex closure method, only when necessary. However, this concept oversimplifies the indication for reconstruction to just wound coverage, ignoring the need for subsequent operation through the same wound as well as for better functional and esthetic restoration. Thus, Gottlieb and Krieger introduced the concept of the reconstructive elevator in 1994, which highlights functional considerations for reconstruction.[12] However, with improved understanding of microsurgical anatomy and advances in surgical technique and tools, surgeons have even more options at their fingertips to restore form and function. Both the concept of the reconstructive ladder and the reconstructive elevator are too simple and rigid to guide decision making. Reconstructive plans are based on multiple factors such as defect location, timing of surgery, patient prognosis, surgeon's skills, and available resources. While some have proposed new metaphors such as the reconstructive grid or matrix to aid in decision making, they inhibit intuition and are difficult to adopt.[11]

Chimeric Flaps

The chimeric flap is another area that has been riddled with misunderstanding and ambiguous terminology. This is partially due to the fact that the idea of combined flap has been introduced since the 1980s, predating studies on microvasculature anatomy and skin vessels.[13] Thus, adjectives such as combined, compound, conjoined, and chimeric have all been used to describe flaps with multiple vascular territories and tissue types.[14] The senior author (FCW) advocates for simplifying the terminology by adopting a definition of chimeric flap that is based on the natural anatomy. A flap is classified as a chimeric flap if it contains 2 or more types of tissues that are different, each tissue component must have a defined pedicle with an independent blood supply, and their pedicles are naturally linked. Some examples of chimeric flap include an ALT flap with an independent vessel that perfuses the vastus lateralis or a fibula flap with a skin paddle and soleus muscle (see **Fig. 2**).

Chimeric flaps are useful for reconstructing composite defects, particularly those that require a 3-dimensional reconstruction or additional volume such as compound defects of the mandible and the maxilla. Furthermore, chimeric flaps may be used instead of double flaps. In such cases, a major advantage of using a chimeric flap is that it only requires 1 donor site and 1 set of recipient vessels. Some of the commonly vascular systems for harvesting chimeric flaps include the lateral circumflex femoral vessels (**Fig. 4**), the peroneal artery vessels, the subscapular vessels, and the uperficial and deep iliac systems. Overall, lower extremity donor sites are preferred because they allow for a 2-team approach, have long pedicles,

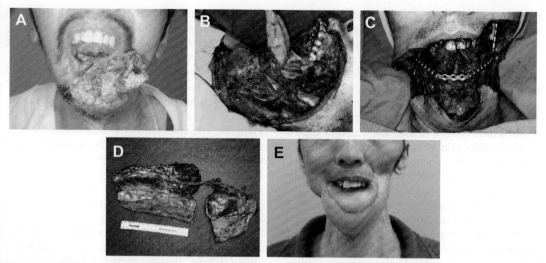

Fig. 4. (*A*) Extensive cancer involvement in the lower lip, chin, and mandible. (*B*) Appearance after cancer excision. (*C*) Mandibular defect stabilized with reconstruction plate. (*D*) Both intraoral and external face reconstructed with an ALT myocutaneous flap and a tensor fascia lata myocutaneous flap from the same source vessel. (*E*) Follow-up appearance at vascularized fibula shall be scheduled for mandibular reconstruction.

and allow for harvest of multiple muddles and large skin territories with minimal donor site morbidity.

Chimeric flaps are more challenging to harvest and inset; thus, surgeons should start with the donor site he or she is most familiar with. The pedicle to each tissue needs to be meticulously dissected and care should be taken to preserve pedicle length. Insetting the chimeric flap may be particularly difficult. Different tissue components should be used to reconstruction different subunits of the defect. For instance, a single large tissue component should not be used for simultaneous reconstruction of both a static and mobile structure. Each tissue component should be inset carefully to ensure that that the pedicle is not twisted or compressed. If any portion of the flap needs to be passed through a tunnel, ensure adequate space in the tunnel before inset—generally, the authors recommend at least 2 finger-breadth width. The more tissue component included in the chimeric flap, the more complex the inset. At the authors' institute, the general preference is to inset the flap before performing the microvascular anastomosis. Thus, it is important to reassess and monitor each tissue component and its pedicle after anastomosis of the main pedicle. In summary, reconstructions using chimeric flaps are very challenging and require careful preoperative planning (see **Fig. 4**).

Perforator Flaps with Multiple Skin Paddles

One of the challenges of oromandibular reconstruction is the involvement of multiple soft-tissue soft units. Defects are often full thickness—involving

both intraoral and extraoral soft-tissue subunits—or involve both the maxillary and mandibular surfaces or gingival sulcus. Proper restoration of form cannot be achieved by simply folding a flap. The ability to sustain multiple skin paddles on a single pedicle affords more versatility and therefore more elegant reconstructive options. Several techniques have been described to create multiple skin paddles. The earliest claim of "double skin paddle" was quite misleading; instead of creating 2 independent skin paddles with 2 independent perfusing vessels, a central skin bridge was de-epithelialized to create 2 skin paddles.[15] This technique preserves the dermal plexus and does not require the identification of multiple perforators.[15] However, the maintenance of the dermis bridge limits the arch rotation around each terminal vessel.[16] Additionally, the de-epithelized skin bridge portion may be too bulky to pass through a tunnel separating the 2 defects. The more versatile option—anatomy permitting—is to design a flap with 2 or more skin perfusing vessels with pedicles that join proximally.[17] This way, each skin paddle has a greater arch of rotation and be inset more independently. Nevertheless, it is important to be conscientious of the tension and compression of each pedicle vessel during flap inset.

Thinning and Shaping Perforator Flaps

Going beyond simply covering defects, further refining reconstruction requires tailoring each flap to the defects' size and thickness. The more conservative approach is to perform flap thinning at a second stage (often several weeks or even months after the index surgery). This is not only safer from a flap perfusion standpoint but mitigates over-debulking the flap as both scar contracture and radiation will reduce the size of the initial flap.

However, better understanding of the anatomic structure of blood vessels has enabled surgeons to perform perforator flap thinning and shaping in a single stage. Typically, flap thinning involves removing the fat located deep to the superficial fascia, which consist of Camper's and Scarpa's fascia. Certain skin vessels are more amenable to thinning as the branching and arborization happens in the in the superficial adipofascial layer, or Camper's fascia.[18]

The most discussed flap for thinning is the ALT flap. According to Nakajima's classification, lateral circumflex femoral artery is a type III artery and not amenable to thinning without jeopardizing vascularity.[18,19] This is consistent with cadaveric studies of the ALT flap that showed that the suprafascial plexus along the deep fascia and is connected to the subdermal plexus.[20] However, several clinical studies have also demonstrated successful thinning of the ALT flap during elevation, especially when 1 to 2 cm cuff of soft tissue is preserved around the perforators.[21,22] Ultimately, the ability to elegantly shape and thin a perforator flap is a combination of anatomic awareness and delicate surgical technique to carefully perform intra-flap dissection of microscopic vessels.

In some limited applications, such as ear reconstruction and facial burn resurfacing, dermal perforator flaps may be indicated. Advanced imaging of the dermal and subdermal plexus demonstrates the existence of up to 3 dermal plexus in super thin flaps with pure skin perforators penetrating the dermis and subdermal plexus.[23] Dermal perforator flaps include a perforating vessel and the subcutaneous tissue around the perforator and pedicle.[24] With the aid of ultra-high-frequency ultrasound (70 MHz), small ($\geq$0.5 mm diameter) direct dermal perforators can be visualized and dissected as a freestyle super thin flap of less than 1 mm thickness[23] However, the size of the vessel in the subdermal plexus is quite small and becomes less reliable; thus, only small flaps can be reliably elevated in this fashion.

Free-Style Elevation of Perforator Flaps

One of the biggest limitations of the current free flaps for head and neck reconstruction is poor skin color, texture, and thickness match.[25] Having access to more donor sites in the body enables the surgeon to select for suitable skin-free flaps for each application. The free-style free flap was first described by Mardini and Wei in 2003 for thigh-based skin flaps.[26] Instead of harvesting one of

the described skin flaps, a flap can be designed around any sizable skin perforator. First, the desired donor site is selected, and Doppler is used to confirm the presence of a vessel superficial to the deep fascia. Generally, larger diameter perforators have more audible Doppler signal.[27] A flap is designed around the identified vessel. Through the exploratory incision, the vessel is identified and dissected. The size of the flap can be determined by the size of the vessel, the volume of tissue, and arborization of vessels in the flap. The freestyle skin flap technique is even more useful for pedicled flaps. The intramuscular pedicle dissection can lengthen the arc of rotation and increase the reach of advancement.

Free style perforator flap is a versatile technique where any site can be selected as potential donor sites for flaps, thereby providing better matches for skin thickness, depth, skin color match, and texture. This is particularly useful for defect where only a small or moderate sized flap is needed. However, one disadvantage of the freestyle perforator flap technique is the unpredictability of the pedicle length and its caliber, which in turn can limit the dimensions of the flap.

FUTURE DEVELOPMENT
Small Recipient Vessels

Modern medicine has revolutionized the mortality and morbidity of head and neck cancers. Unfortunately, the head and neck cancer survivors are also the ones most at risk for recurrence or second primaries, often presenting for secondary, tertiary, even quaternary resections that require reconstruction. Each reconstruction becomes increasingly more challenging as the reconstructive surgeon must overcome the effects of radiation, fibrosis, and an fewer option for recipient vessels. Microsurgical techniques have not only increased the surgeon's armamentarium of flaps, but also expand the repertoire of available recipient vessels. This concept has been coined "perforator-to-perforator" flaps and while the authors do not agree with the terminology, the physiology is sound and should be applied in head and neck reconstruction.

"Perforator-to-perforator" anastomosis refers to anastomosis to recipient vessels ranging from 0.3 to 0.8 mm. While there is a plethora of reports on using this technique for lower extremity reconstruction,[28] the adaption for head and neck reconstruction is more scarce.[29] Advantages of using these small superficial vessels as recipient vessels are straightforward: they are abundant; they require less dissection and therefore less operative time; and they do not require sacrifice of a major vessel which is important in a vessel-depleted neck.

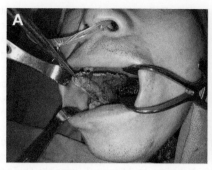
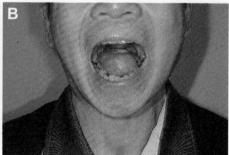

Fig. 5. Tongue. (*A*) Appearance after hemiglossectomy. (*B*) Appearance of ALT reconstructed tongue at 1 year postoperation.

However, small recipient vessels are also challenging to manage, and real-time assessment of flow is critical. In fact, Hong and colleagues emphasizes that that assessment of the recipient small vessel, particularly vessels 0.3 to 0.4 mm, should be performed prior to transecting the donor flap.[28] Furthermore, performing such anastomosis is technically demanding, often requiring smaller microsutures (12-0 nylon or smaller) and microneedles (30–50 μm). Nevertheless, many studies have demonstrated flap success rates equal to conventional microsurgical techniques.[28,29]

Application of Imaging Technology in Microsurgery

The past 3 decades of anatomic studies and clinical studies have irrefutably proven the safety and versatility of perforators flaps. The new frontier of soft tissue coverage is to further the safety, efficacy, cost-effectiveness, and restore esthetic such as skin color match and cosmetic subunits. To this end, many new imaging technologies have been introduced to enhance visualization of tiny structures. Ultra-high-frequency ultrasound is one of the most discussed emerging technologies in the literature. With 48 and 70 MHz linear probes, a surgeon can visualize structure as small as 30 μm[23,30] Clinically, perforators visualized on ultra-high-frequency ultrasound are well correlated with perforators on dissection.[30] Proof of concept studies have demonstrated some benefit using ultra-high-frequency ultrasound to improve surgical planning and preoperative perforator selection for raising thin and ultra-thin flaps.[30]

Another emerging technology with promising results is intraoperative microscope-integrated laser tomography which would allow for more objective evaluation of microsurgical anastomosis.[31] Similarly, intraoperative use of indocyanine green and fluorescence imaging allows the surgeon to objectively assess flap perfusion immediately following completion of flap pedicle dissection and after

microsurgical anastomosis.[32] Indocyanine green angiography can detect vasculature less than 0.2 mm in diameter.[32] These tools are designed to help the surgeons take the guesswork out of microsurgery.

SUMMARY

Since their introduction in the late 1980s, perforator flaps have gradually been adopted by head and neck surgeons for reconstruction of soft tissue defects. While local adjacent tissue may also be used for reconstruction—and offer better skin match—there are still concerns about "field of cancerization," and therefore should be avoided, especially in the setting of oral squamous cell carcinoma. Many flaps have been described, but only several have become workhorse flaps for head and neck reconstruction including the ALT flap, AMT flap, PAP, and medial sural artery perforator (MSAP) flap. Mastery of intramuscular dissection technique of these flaps will cover most head and neck defects (**Fig. 5**). Beyond the fundamentals of flap elevation, further understanding of skin flap microvascular anatomy allows for more sophisticated shaping and further refinement.

CLINICS CARE POINTS

- Microsurgical free flaps have become the standard of care for reconstructing composite head and neck defects.

- Mastery of the perforator flap, especially the ALT flap's intramuscular dissection enables the surgeon to elevate almost any soft tissue flap needed for coverage of most head and neck defects.

- New imaging technology and improved understanding of skin microvasculature can further refine the safety and outcome of soft tissue reconstruction.

DISCLOSURE

The authors have no relevant or material financial that relates to the research described in this paper.

REFERENCES

1. Milton SH. Pedicled skin-flaps: the fallacy of the length: width ratio. Br J Surg 1970;57(7):502–8.
2. Taylor GI, Palmer JH. The vascular territories (angiosomes) of the body: experimental study and clinical applications. Br J Plast Surg 1987;40(2):113–41.
3. Koshima I, Soeda S. Inferior epigastric artery skin flaps without rectus abdominis muscle. Br J Plast Surg 1989;42(6):645–8.
4. Nakajima H, Fujino T, Adachi S. A new concept of vascular supply to the skin and classification of skin flaps according to their vascularization. Ann Plast Surg 1986;16(1):1.
5. Blondeel PN, Van Landuyt KHI, Monstrey SJM, et al. The "Gent" consensus on perforator flap terminology: preliminary definitions. Plast Reconstr Surg 2003;112(5):1378–83 [quiz 1383, 1516; discussion 1384-1387].
6. Song YG, zhang Chen G, liang Song Y. The free thigh flap: a new free flap concept based on the septocutaneous artery. Br J Plast Surg 1984;37(2): 149–59.
7. Lutz BS, Wei FC. Microsurgical workhorse flaps in head and neck reconstruction. Clin Plast Surg 2005;32(3):421–30, vii.
8. Lin SJ, Butler CE. Subtotal thigh flap and bioprosthetic mesh reconstruction for large, composite abdominal wall defects. Plast Reconstr Surg 2010; 125(4):1146–56.
9. Kimata Y, Uchiyama K, Ebihara S, et al. Anterolateral thigh flap donor-site complications and morbidity. Plast Reconstr Surg 2000;106(3):584.
10. Yu P. Inverse relationship of the anterolateral and anteromedial thigh flap perforator anatomy. J Reconstr Microsurg 2014;30(7):463–8.
11. Hallock GG. The reconstructive toolbox. Arch Plast Surg 2023;50(4):331–4.
12. Gottlieb LJ, Krieger LM. From the reconstructive ladder to the reconstructive elevator. Plast Reconstr Surg 1994;93(7):1503.
13. Harii K, Iwaya T, Kawaguchi N. Combination myocutaneous flap and microvascular free flap. Plast Reconstr Surg 1981;68(5):700.
14. Hallock GG. The complete nomenclature for combined perforator flaps. Plast Reconstr Surg 2011; 127(4):1720–9.
15. Jones NF, Vögelin E, Markowitz BL, et al. Reconstruction of composite through-and-through mandibular defects with a double-skin paddle fibular osteocutaneous flap. Plast Reconstr Surg 2003;112(3):758.
16. Kubo T, Osaki Y, Hattori R, et al. Reconstruction of through-and-through oromandibular defects by the double-skin paddle fibula osteocutaneous flap: Can the skin paddle always be divided? J Plast Surg Hand Surg 2013;47(1):46–9.
17. Chang EI, Yu P. Prospective series of reconstruction of complex composite mandibulectomy defects with double island free fibula flap. J Surg Oncol 2017; 116(2):258–62.
18. Park SO, Chang H, Imanishi N. Anatomic basis for flap thinning. Arch Plast Surg 2018;45(4):298–303.
19. Nakajima H, Minabe T, Imanishi N. Three-dimensional analysis and classification of arteries in the skin and subcutaneous adipofascial tissue by computer graphics imaging. Plast Reconstr Surg 1998; 102(3):748–60.
20. Schaverien M, Saint-Cyr M, Arbique G, et al. Three- and four-dimensional computed tomographic angiography and venography of the anterolateral thigh perforator flap. Plast Reconstr Surg 2008;121(5): 1685.
21. Nojima K, Brown SA, Acikel C, et al. Defining vascular supply and territory of thinned perforator flaps: part i. anterolateral thigh perforator flap. Plast Reconstr Surg 2005;116(1):182.
22. Prasetyono TO, Bangun K, Buchari FB, et al. Practical considerations for perforator flap thinning procedures revisited. Arch Plast Surg 2014;41(6):693–701.
23. Yoshimatsu H, Hayashi A, Yamamoto T, et al. Visualization of the "Intradermal Plexus" Using Ultrasonography in the Dermis Flap: A Step beyond Perforator Flaps. Plast Reconstr Surg Glob Open 2019;7(11): e2411.
24. Narushima M, Yamasoba T, Iida T, et al. Pure skin perforator flaps: the anatomical vascularity of the superthin flap. Plast Reconstr Surg 2018;142(3): 351e.
25. Menick FJ. Facial reconstruction with local and distant tissue: the interface of aesthetic and reconstructive surgery. Plast Reconstr Surg 1998;102(5):1424.
26. Mardini S, Tsai FC, Wei FC. The thigh as a model for free style free flaps. Clin Plast Surg 2003;30(3): 473–80.
27. Blondeel PN, Beyens G, Verhaeghe R, et al. Doppler flowmetry in the planning of perforator flaps. Br J Plast Surg 1998;51(3):202–9.
28. Hong JP. The use of supermicrosurgery in lower extremity reconstruction: the next step in evolution. Plast Reconstr Surg 2009;123(1):230.
29. MacKenzie A, Dhoot A, Rehman U, et al. Use of supermicrosurgery in craniofacial and head and neck soft tissue reconstruction: a systematic review of the literature and meta-analysis. Br J Oral Maxillofac Surg 2024;62(2):140–9.
30. Visconti G, Bianchi A, Hayashi A, et al. Pure skin perforator flap direct elevation above the subdermal plane using preoperative ultra-high frequency

ultrasound planning: A proof of concept. J Plast Reconstr Aesthetic Surg 2019;72(10):1700–38.

31. Hayashi A, Yoshimatsu H, Visconti G, et al. Intraoperative real-time visualization of the lymphatic vessels using microscope-integrated laser tomography. J Reconstr Microsurg 2021;37(5):427–35.

32. Ludolph I, Horch RE, Arkudas A, et al. Enhancing safety in reconstructive microsurgery using intraoperative indocyanine green angiography. Front Surg 2019;6. Available at: https://www.frontiersin.org/articles/10.3389/fsurg.2019.00039. [Accessed 14 January 2024].

Functional Perspectives in Tongue Reconstruction Based on Perforator Free Flap

Jong Woo Choi, MD, PhD, MMM*, Young Chul Kim, MD

KEYWORDS

- Tongue • Dynamic reconstruction • Function • Swallowing • Speech

KEY POINTS

- Successful functional tongue reconstruction requires not only advancements in surgical techniques but also meticulous coordination with oncological treatments.
- It is crucial to meticulously tailor the choice of flap, adjust flap volume, and determine flap placement to optimize postoperative functionality.
- Restoring the ideal motion vector is essential for maximizing the functional results in dynamic tongue reconstruction using motor-innervated free flaps.

INTRODUCTION

Tongue reconstruction following oncological resection presents a significant challenge in the head and neck surgery, demanding an approach that balances anatomic restoration with the preservation of functions including speech, swallowing, and mastication.[1] Innovations in microsurgical techniques, particularly the perforator flap concept, have markedly enhanced flap selection, facilitating tailored reconstructive solutions for tongue defects.[2,3] However, the intricate anatomy of the tongue, and its critical role in physiologic functions, demands comprehensive understanding of the structural and functional consequences of different reconstructive strategies.

This article investigates the comprehensive aspects of tongue reconstruction, emphasizing the critical role of functional tongue reconstruction. It addresses the significance of defect classification, establishing a strategic foundation for reconstruction, and delves into the detailed selection of flap characteristics, aiming to achieve both anatomic integrity and functional normalcy. Further, the article explores into the advancements in reconstructive techniques, for optimizing flap volume and tailoring flap shape and inset to closely replicate the tongue's 3-dimensional (3D) structure.

Advancements in functional tongue reconstruction extend to dynamic reconstruction, leveraging motor-innervated flaps to closely mimic the tongue's muscular actions.[4–6] Compared with traditional methods using fasciocutaneous flaps, this approach aims to restore the tongue dynamics, crucial for effective swallowing and speech. By examining these advancements in dynamic methods, including the importance of careful flap selection, technical details, and functional benefits of motor-innervated free flaps, this review aims to encapsulate the current state of the art in functional tongue reconstruction.

KEY CONSIDERATION IN FUNCTIONAL TONGUE RECONSTRUCTION

Several key considerations distinguish tongue reconstruction from other reconstructive procedures within the oral cavity.[1,7] First, prompt and complication-free wound healing in the neo-tongue is crucial to avoid delaying any necessary postoperative radiation therapy, which can escalate the risk of cancer recurrence and mortality.[8]

Department of Plastic and Reconstructive Surgery, University of Ulsan College of Medicine, Asan Medical Center, 88, Olympic-ro 43-gil, SongPa-Gu, Seoul 05505, Korea
* Corresponding author.
E-mail address: pschoi@amc.seoul.kr

Oral Maxillofacial Surg Clin N Am 36 (2024) 435–449
https://doi.org/10.1016/j.coms.2024.07.011
1042-3699/24/© 2024 Elsevier Inc. All rights reserved, including those for text and data mining, AI training, and similar technologies.

Secondly, careful consideration of functional mobility of the neo-tongue is essential during flap selection and defect volume assessment. Effective functional reconstruction hinges on preserving tongue mobility for speech and swallowing, alongside ensuring adequate volume for palatal contact.[9] Thirdly, the volume and shape of the reconstructed neo-tongue are critical. The volume of the chosen flap significantly influences swallowing efficiency, fills dead space, and aids in preventing aspiration by channeling food and saliva away from the airway.[10,11] Fourth, in cases involving concurrent defects in other oropharyngeal structures, the preoperative volume of the tongue and intended postoperative volume should guide flap selection, which in turn, impacts the functional outcomes of the neo-tongue.[12] Lastly, maintaining oral and oropharyngeal swallowing and speech functions remains the primary goal, as the tongue is essential for these activities.[13] The success of tongue reconstruction depends on addressing these interrelated considerations, each contributing to the overall rehabilitative outcome.

DEFECT CLASSIFICATION

A systematic classification is essential to methodically identify intraoral defects arising from tongue cancer. These defects are typically sequalae of surgical tumor resection, with the majority of lingual malignancies manifesting along the lateral border of the anterior two-thirds of the tongue.[14] This distribution shows no preference for laterality, with unilateral presentation being the most common. Surgical removal of tongue tumors, known as glossectomy, forms the basis for categorizing the resultant defects. Ansarin and colleagues devised a detailed classification, ranging from mucosectomy to partial and hemiglossectomy of varying extents, to subtotal and total glossectomy, based on the anatomic and functional impact of the resection.[15] Specifically, partial glossectomy involves the resection of less than one-third of the tongue, hemiglossectomy pertains to the removal of one-third to half, subtotal glossectomy encompasses the excision of half to three-quarters, and total glossectomy denotes complete removal of the tongue[6] (**Fig. 1**).

Additional refinement of this classification incorporates volumetric and locational aspects of the defects. For instance, Bhattacharya and colleagues adhered to the aforementioned volumetric categories while introducing locational codes: L for lateral oral tongue defects, potentially including the tongue base; T for tip defects anterior to the frenulum's attachment; and S for sulcal and floor of the mouth defects.[16] Mannelli and colleagues's functional subunit system further delineates defects based on unilateral presence, extent over one-third of the mobile tongue, involvement of the tongue base, and any association with the floor of the mouth, categorizing them into 5 distinct types.[17]

These classification systems underscore the complexity and variability of tongue cancer-related defects, implicating numerous adjacent anatomic structures in the reconstructive process. Therefore, the reconstructive surgeon must accurately identify each specific intraoral defect in relation to the original anatomic feature, utilizing these classification systems to inform their approach. For instance, Butler and colleagues proposed a tri-laminar principle for classifying oral cavity defects, assigning numeric and letter codes to indicate the extent of the defect and structures involved.[18] Liu and colleagues introduced a 6-zone classification, focusing on the horizontal and vertical dimensions of oral cavity structures affected by the defect, thereby facilitating the selection of reconstructive options for optimal functional outcomes.[19] The head and neck defect classification system proposed by Choi and colleagues organizes defects into zones, each further divided into 3 subzones (A, B, and C) to comprehensively describe the location and extent of resection-associated defects. This system facilitates precise communication and planning for reconstructive surgery by providing a standardized framework for identifying defects (**Table 1**).

ANATOMIC AND FUNCTIONAL CONSIDERATION
Flap Volume

Optimizing neo-tongue volume by focusing on achieving palatal contact to improve speech and swallowing is crucial for enhancing the functional outcomes of tongue reconstruction.[9–11] For defects affecting up to two-thirds of the tongue, using a thin, pliable flap that provides sufficient bulk to fill dead space with adequate width to avoid tethering the neo-tongue tip to the floor of the mouth is advisable.[20] For more extensive resection, such as total tongue resection, larger flaps are necessary to maximize functional outcomes. In such cases, a convex rather than concave neo-tongue shape is preferred to mitigate salivary pooling and aspiration risks.[21]

Historically, a protuberant neo-tongue volume and shape, extending above the teeth level, were considered ideal. A 4-point scoring system is used to assess the achievement of optimal tongue geometry.[22] In this system, a score of 1

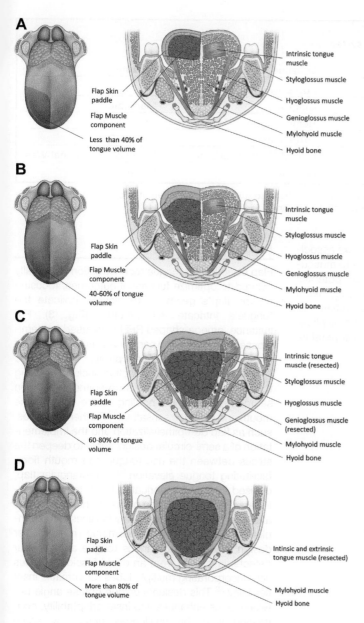

A

Intrinsic tongue muscle
Styloglossus muscle
Hyoglossus muscle
Genioglossus muscle
Mylohyoid muscle
Hyoid bone

Flap Skin paddle
Flap Muscle component
Less than 40% of tongue volume

B

Intrinsic tongue muscle
Styloglossus muscle
Hyoglossus muscle
Genioglossus muscle
Mylohyoid muscle
Hyoid bone

Flap Skin paddle
Flap Muscle component
40-60% of tongue volume

C

Intrinsic tongue muscle (resected)
Styloglossus muscle
Hyoglossus muscle
Genioglossus muscle (resected)
Mylohyoid muscle
Hyoid bone

Flap Skin paddle
Flap Muscle component
60-80% of tongue volume

D

Intinsic and extrinsic tongue muscle (resected)
Mylohyoid muscle
Hyoid bone

Flap Skin paddle
Flap Muscle component
More than 80% of tongue volume

Fig. 1. Schematic representation of the dynamic reconstruction method, illustrating the positioning of cutaneous and muscle components for different extents of glossectomy (*A*) Partial tongue reconstruction involves the resection of less than one-third of the tongue. (*B*) Hemi-tongue reconstruction covers the removal of one-third to half of the tongue. (*C*) Subtotal reconstruction encompasses the excision of half to three-quarters of the tongue. (*D*) Total or near-total tongue reconstruction denotes the complete removal of the tongue. (*From* Refs.[5,6])

indicates a tongue that is depressed, concave, and situated below the upper mandibular margin, signifying a less ideal outcome. A score of 2 is assigned to a tongue that is level with the mandible and teeth, representing an intermediate condition. A score of 3 denotes a semi-protuberant, convex tongue that enables the soft palate to be seen and extends above the upper edge of the teeth, approximating the desired geometry. Lastly, a score of 4 describes a protuberant, convex tongue that obscures the view of the oropharynx, considered the optimal reconstructive outcome. This scoring system guides the reconstruction process toward achieving

tongue geometry conducive to improved speech and swallowing functions (**Fig. 2**).

Recent technological advancements have enabled postoperative 3D evaluations of the flap and neo-tongue volume, yielding more accurate and consistent assessments for functional outcomes.[23] Maintaining the neo-tongue volume postoperatively remains a challenge owing to the effects of patient factors (eg, age), postoperative radiation, and flap characteristics on volume retention. Studies have observed significant volume reduction (11%–44%) in patients receiving postoperative radiation.[24,25] Fasciocutaneous flaps, akin to radial forearm free flaps (RFFFs)

Table 1
Head and neck defect classification system

Zone	Subzone A	Subzone B	Subzone C
1	Skin	Buccal Mucosa	Lip
2	Floor of the Mouth	Gingiva	Mandible
3	Partial Tongue	Hemi-Tongue	Total Tongue
4	Tonsil	Soft Palate	Tongue Base
5	Anterior Pharyngeal Wall	Lateral Pharyngeal Wall	Posterior Pharyngeal Wall
6	Hard Palate	Maxilla	Orbit

This system not only aids in the surgical planning process but also supports the selection of appropriate reconstructive techniques to achieve optimal functional and esthetic outcomes.

and anterolateral thigh (ALT) free flaps, are associated with lesser volume loss compared to musculocutaneous flaps.[26] To counteract potential volume loss and ensure functional efficacy, flaps should be oversized by 20% to 30% relative to the defect, with some recommending a multiplication factor of 1.4 for flap volume if postoperative radiation is anticipated.[22,24,25,27]

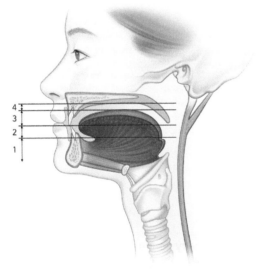

Fig. 2. Tongue volume evaluation Volume Score (1–4); Score 4, protuberant (obscures the oropharynx view); Score 3, semi-protuberant (convex, yet allows soft palate visibility, with the tongue positioned above the upper margin of the lower teeth); Score 2, flat (neither convex nor concave, positioning the tongue between the upper margin of the lower teeth and the mandible); and Score 1, depressed (concave, placing the tongue below the upper margin of the mandible). (Redrawn from Yun IS, Lee DW, Lee WJ, Lew DH, Choi EC, Rah DK. Correlation of neotongue volume changes with functional outcomes after long-term follow-up of total glossectomy. The Journal of Craniofacial Surgery. Jan 2010;21(1):111-6.)

Flap Shape and Inset

Flap selection for tongue reconstruction is critically tailored to optimize functional outcomes, focusing on the flap's geometry to closely replicate the tongue's intricate 3D structure (**Fig. 3**). For instance, omega-shaped RFFFs are used for hemiglossectomy, featuring narrow waists that resemble the tongue's cross-sectional profile.[28] Techniques to enhance tongue tip function include rotating the flap tip combined with a de-epithelialized skin segment to minimize pooling in the floor of the mouth and enhance sensation.[29] Further strategies, such as flap de-epithelialization and the implementation of a semi-circular design, serve to deepen the sulcus between the neo-tongue and mouth floor, facilitating tongue elevation.[30] A rectangular flap, devised from a pre-fabricated RFFF template, delineates clear boundaries between the neo-tongue and mouth floor, guided by tension lines in the template.[31] Additionally, a geometric multi-lobular design, adaptable to various tongue and tonsillar defects, is crafted from an ovoid fasciocutaneous flap, incorporating multiple lobes for versatile inset flexibility.[32] This design's unique obtuse angle between lobes enhances flap inset adaptability, contrasting with the challenges posed by acute angles in positioning.

For extensive reconstructions, such as total and subtotal glossectomy, flap designs prioritize both bulk and mobility, tailored to the specific flap type (see **Fig. 3**). For instance, beavertail extensions in RFFFs serve a dual purpose: covering adjacent soft tissue defects and providing volume augmentation through de-epithelialization.[33,34] Similarly, innovative ALT flap designs have been innovatively designed from mushroom-shaped configurations with de-epithelialized islands for protuberance to "sushi roll" and pentagonal musculocutaneous designs for enhanced longitudinal projection and a sloping cross-sectional profile.[35,36] For individuals with a lower body mass

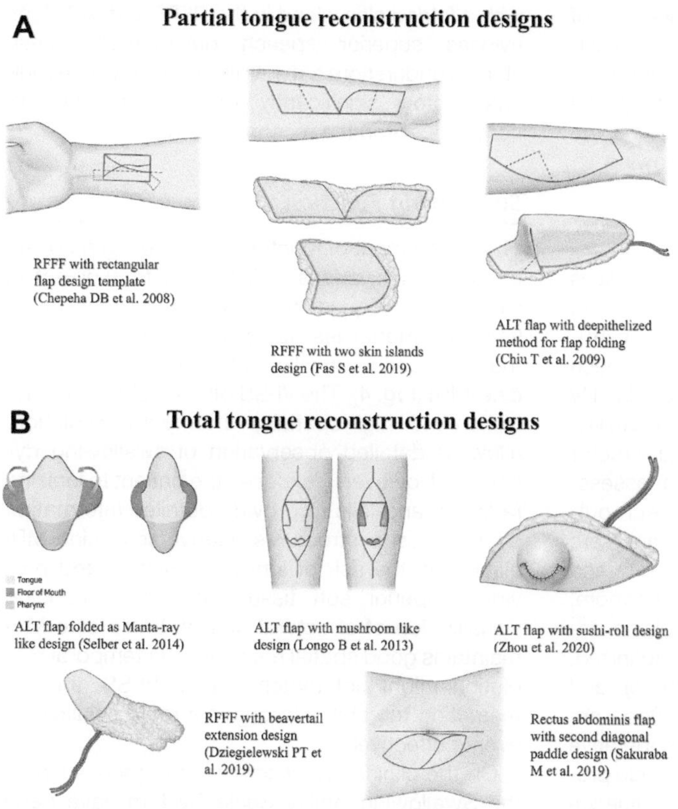

A   Partial tongue reconstruction designs

RFFF with rectangular
flap design template
(Chepeha DB et al. 2008)

RFFF with two skin islands
design (Fas S et al. 2019)

ALT flap with deepithelized
method for flap folding
(Chiu T et al. 2009)

B   Total tongue reconstruction designs

Tongue
Floor of Mouth
Pharynx

ALT flap folded as Manta-ray
like design (Selber et al. 2014)

ALT flap with mushroom like
design (Longo B et al. 2013)

ALT flap with sushi-roll design
(Zhou et al. 2020)

RFFF with beavertail
extension design
(Dziegielewski PT et
al. 2019)

Rectus abdominis flap
with second diagonal
paddle design (Sakuraba
M et al. 2019)

Fig. 3. Different flap designs vary according to the type of flap and the extent of the tongue resection defect. (*A*) Diverse designs for partial tongue reconstruction for both the radial forearm free flap (RFFF) and the anterolateral thigh (ALT) flap. (*B*) Total and subtotal tongue reconstruction designs with geometric designs incorporated in the RFF, ALT, and rectus abdominis musculocutaneous flaps. (*From* Choi JW, Alshomer F, Kim YC. Evolution and current status of microsurgical tongue reconstruction, part II. Archives of craniofacial surgery. Oct 2022;23(5):193-204. https://doi.org/10.7181/acfs.2022.00857.)

index, a dual-skin island vertical rectus abdominis musculocutaneous flap can offer the necessary bulk and outer structure.[37]

Virtual surgical planning and 3D printing technologies have been employed to design customized tongue-shaped flaps, enhancing the precision of reconstructive surgeries. This process involves initial analysis of the tumor's extent via preoperative 0.5-mm 3D computed tomography.[38] Based on this analysis, a specific soft tissue cutting guide tailored to the tongue tumor is created, followed by the fabrication of a post-excisional defect guide to aid in flap harvesting. Although initial proof-of-concept studies have demonstrated the effectiveness of this approach, further research is necessary to assess its effect on patient survival, functional outcomes, and its cost-effectiveness. This innovative method represents a significant advancement in surgical planning, offering potential for more personalized and effective reconstructive outcomes.

Tongue Mobility

The tongue plays a crucial role within the oral cavity, being essential for breathing, speech, and swallowing. Its functionality stems from a sophisticated and delicate morphology comprising various muscular components, specifically, the genioglossus, transversus, verticalis, and superior longitudinal muscle groups.[39] These muscle groups enable a range of movements and contortions across multiple axes, facilitated by interdigitations allowing for both antagonistic and delicate micromotions crucial for the tongue's myriad functions.

Despite advancements in microsurgical reconstructive techniques, replicating a fully mobile neo-tongue that matches the natural tongue's capabilities remains a challenging yet actively pursued goal. The mobility of the reconstructed tongue largely depends on the mobility of the residual tongue post-resection and the transmitted movement from surrounding phalangeal muscles.[40,41] Consequently, the extent of tongue resection is proportional to its effect on the impairment of tongue movement, with tongue base resection considerably limiting movement and impairing residual tongue function.

Various methods have been developed to quantitatively and qualitatively assess tongue mobility, focusing on movements such as protrusion, elevation, depression, lateralization, retroflexion, dorsal elevation, and retraction. These assessments are integral to routine speech and swallowing rehabilitation, providing a quantitative measure of functional outcomes. Additionally, radiologic evaluations of tongue mobility contribute to comprehensive swallowing assessments, underscoring the significance of tongue mobility in determining the functional outcomes for speech and swallowing.[42]

Speech Function

Traditionally, speech assessment encompasses subjective methods, including perceptual and acoustic evaluations. Additionally, objective instruments have been developed to scrutinize speech functionality, assessing speech understandability and intelligibility, reading time and acceptability, articulation errors, diadochokinetic rate, and motor impulse speed and substitution. These assessments focus on their implications for speech outcomes; neo-tongue mobility and protuberance are positively correlated with speech intelligibility and favorable subjective outcomes.[43,44] Furthermore, the repercussions of tumor size and excision defects, leading to tissue loss, have been scrutinized. Advanced stage disease (T3 and above) and excisions affecting the tongue tip or floor are detrimental to speech outcomes.[45] Preoperative and postoperative radiation therapy, alongside preoperative chemotherapy, significantly influence speech functionality, with smoking status and persistent tracheostomy linked to adverse speech outcomes.[46–48]

Studies have not found significant differences in speech functionality among the various flap options, although some suggest marginally better outcomes with RFFFs for lateral oral tongue defect reconstruction, highlighting the influence of flap and defect traits on tongue mobility. For instance, thin, pliable flaps such as RFFFs, with long vascular pedicles, outperform pectoralis major myocutaneous flaps, which are marred by the effects of pedicle tethering and gravity, hindering tongue mobility.[12] The defect location further influences the functional outcomes; deterioration of speech intelligibility occurs in defects encompassing both the anterior oral tongue and tongue base post-reconstruction.[45]

Studies have been evaluated the effect of flap features, including shape and dimensions, on speech outcomes and found that flap length is inversely related to speech articulation and intelligibility.[47] Various flap designs have been proposed to address tongue defects, which impact speech outcomes differently. For instance, the L-shaped modification of the ALT flap skin paddle for hemiglossectomy defect reconstruction yields superior speech outcomes than those of traditional rectangular flaps.[49] Similarly, reducing the flap width

with a folded skin island in the RFFF and ALT flaps evinces superior speech outcomes.[50] These studies underscore a dynamic scenario where multiple factors significantly influence speech outcomes post-tongue reconstruction.

Swallowing Function

The assessment of functional swallowing recovery encompasses various tools ranging from objective clinical techniques to subjective assessment. Objective modalities include the videofluoroscopic modified barium swallow study (VFSS/MBS) and cine-MRI (**Fig. 4**). The VFSS offers real-time visualization with high spatial and temporal resolution, allowing detailed observation of swallowing dynamics. However, it exposes the patient to ionizing radiation and fails to provide detailed information on soft tissue structures. Conversely, cine-MRI eliminates the risk of ionizing radiation and provides superior soft tissue contrast, enhancing visualization of structural details. While cine-MRI maintains good spatial resolution, its temporal resolution might not match that of VFSS, thereby restricting the ability to observe rapid swallowing events effectively.

On the clinical assessment front, tools such as the Swallowing Ability Scale System have been developed to systematically evaluate the efficiency and time necessary for food consumption, given the variation in difficulty based on the physical characteristics of different food types.[51] Other clinical assessment tools, including the Rosenbek Penetration Aspiration Scale, 100-mL water swallow test, Performance Status Scale, and Normalcy of Diet Scale, cover a wide range of evaluations.[52] These tools vary in their approach from measuring the risk of aspiration and penetration to assessing the volume and speed of water swallowing and evaluating the patient's overall ability to return to a normal diet.

Swallowing outcomes are influenced by various factors extending from the period before surgery through the recovery period and beyond. Preoperative adjuvant therapy has been linked to reduced tongue mobility and impaired swallowing.[53] The extent of tongue resection correlates with swallowing recovery; larger resections typically result in poorer functional outcomes.[45] Patients with composite defects, including those requiring mandibulectomy, tend to have worse outcomes compared to those with isolated tongue resection. Kim and colleagues observed that swallowing function undergoes sequential changes during the postoperative period, influenced by time-dependent factors such as adjuvant treatment and disease progression.[5] They found that most patients achieve

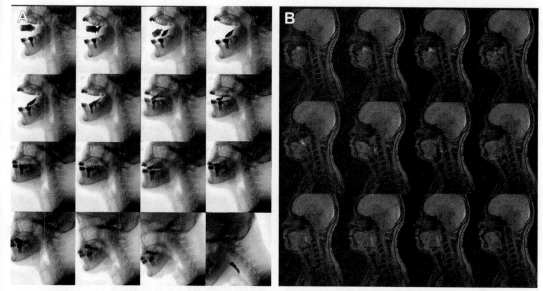

Fig. 4. Lateral view of a VFSS and cine-MRI of a patient who underwent hemiglossectomy reconstruction (*A*) The VFSS offers real-time visualization with high spatial and temporal resolution, allowing detailed observation of swallowing dynamics. However, it exposes the patient to ionizing radiation and lacks detailed information on soft tissue structures. (*B*) Cine-MRI eliminates the risk of ionizing radiation and provides superior soft tissue contrast, enhancing visualization of structural details. While cine-MRI maintains good spatial resolution, its temporal resolution might not match that of VFSS, which could restrict the ability to observe rapid swallowing events effectively. VFSS: videofluoroscopic swallow study.

unrestricted oral intake within 6 months post-surgery, with VFSS/MBS depicting a return to baseline function by 1 year. However, outcomes vary according to the site of resection: tongue base resections are associated with a higher incidence of aspiration and combined oral and tongue base resections show varied recovery timelines.[45]

DYNAMIC TONGUE RECONSTRUCTION

The traditional approach to tongue reconstruction has predominantly utilized fasciocutaneous free flaps, valued for their design flexibility and suitability for adjuvant treatment. However, fasciocutaneous free flaps fundamentally alter the tongue's dynamic nature, converting it into a static entity, thus affecting functionality, especially swallowing. To address these limitations, motor-innervated free flaps have been explored as a dynamic alternative to imitate the muscular action of the native tongue.

Pioneering research with innervated musculocutaneous flaps, such as those derived from the rectus abdominis and gracilis muscles, has shown promising results.[4,6,40,54–58] These muscle transfers not only add volume but also facilitate intimate contact between the reconstructed tongue and remaining oral structures, pivotal for the restoration of swallowing function. Advanced flap designs, including composite or chimeric patterns, further

enhance dynamic reconstruction by providing distinct mobile and static subunits within a single flap, aiding in more complex and functional reconstructions.[6,55] The choice of flap depends on the specific clinical scenario, extent of resection, and individual patient's anatomy and needs.

Conventional Dynamic Tongue Reconstruction Technique

The dynamic tongue reconstruction relies on the use of the gracilis muscle flap; early techniques focused on creating supportive structures and enabling muscle contraction to mimic the tongue's movement. In 2007, Sharma and colleagues introduced gastro omental-dynamic gracilis flaps for near-total glossectomy defects.[56] This technique involved anchoring the gracilis muscle longitudinally to the mandible and hyoid bone, complemented by anastomosis to the hypoglossal nerve and incorporation of gastric mucosa to form the tongue surface. They found that the cross-sectional diameter of the gracilis muscle was similar to that of the normal tongue, allowing it to be tailored to the necessary length and fit comfortably within the constrained space of the mandibular arch (**Fig. 5**).

Calabrese and colleagues (2011) introduced the transverse myocutaneous gracilis flap in 10 patients with partial or total glossectomy.[58] In this technique,

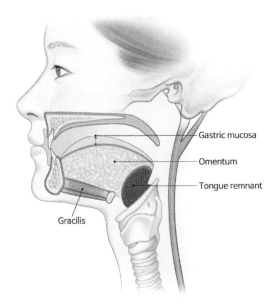

Fig. 5. Sharma's method for dynamic tongue reconstruction. The gracilis muscle is anchored between mandible and hyoid and the gastric mucosa is incorporated to recreate the tongue surface. (Redrawn from Sharma M, Iyer S, Kuriakose MA, et al. Functional reconstruction of near total glossectomy defects using composite gastro-omental-dynamic gracilis flaps. Journal of Plastic, Reconstructive & Aesthetic Surgery: JPRAS. Oct 2009;62(10):1277-80. doi:10.1016/j.bjps.2007.10.092.)

the gracilis muscle is aligned longitudinally between the mandibular body and hyoid bone to establish a supportive sling. The muscle's distal segment is folded to reconstruct either the remaining section of the floor of the mouth or tip of the tongue. The hyoid bone is secured by suspending it from the mandibular ramus laterally with 2 absorbable sutures. This approach effectively provides the necessary bulk for the reconstructed neo-tongue, with its ribbon-like configuration conducive to creating an ideal structure for the floor of the mouth (**Fig. 6**).

Another technique explored by Righini and colleagues (2018) involves the use of an innervated gracilis myocutaneous flap in patients undergoing total glossectomy with laryngeal preservation. In their method, the flap is transversely positioned to create a sling, facilitating the elevation of the neo-tongue via active muscle contraction.[57] Subsequently, it is securely attached with direct sutures to the mandible and laryngeal cartilage or to the preserved hyoid bone. Once transplanted and secured between the mandible's posterior border and hyoid bone, its contraction shifts from an isotonic to isometric mode. This adjustment allows the muscle to bulge and mimic the thrusting action of the tongue, effectively propelling the food bolus into the pharynx and elevating the larynx through isotonic contraction, thus replicating the swallowing process.

Despite their effectiveness, these methods are constrained by the limitations of musculocutaneous flaps, which struggle to replicate the tongue's 3D structure and motion vectors of its dynamic movements.

Introduction of Chimeric Flaps in Dynamic Tongue Reconstruction

The development and introduction of chimeric flaps have marked a significant shift in the approach to tongue reconstruction, aiming to address the shortcomings of traditional musculocutaneous flaps. These techniques offer the advantage of separately incorporating skin paddles and muscle components, enabling 3D reconstruction and flexible vector adjustment.

Ozkan and colleagues discussed the use of a chimeric ALT flap with sensory and motor innervation for reconstructing total or subtotal glossectomy defects.[55] The vastus lateralis muscle (VLM) is affixed to the posterior aspect of the mandible through drill holes. It is then anchored anteromedially to the hyoid bone using

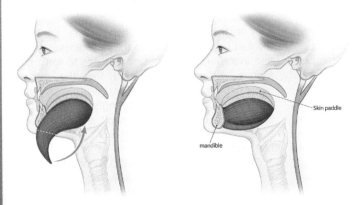

Fig. 6. Calabrese's method for dynamic tongue reconstruction. The gracilis muscle is aligned longitudinally between the mandibular body and the hyoid bone, forming a supportive sling. Its distal part is folded to rebuild either the floor of the mouth or the tongue's tip. (Redrawn from Calabrese L, Saito A, Navach V, et al. Tongue reconstruction with the gracilis myocutaneous free flap. Microsurgery. Jul 2011;31(5):355-9. doi:10.1002/micr. 20885.)

circumferential suturing around the hyoid body. This innovative approach enables the VLM to assume the functional roles traditionally performed by the swallowing muscles, including the geniohyoid, anterior belly of the digastric, mylohyoid, and genioglossus muscles. The fasciocutaneous sections of the flap are then sutured together (or folded onto themselves) to sculpt a tongue-like shape with a defined narrow waist. This approach preserves native tongue characteristics (bulk, mobility, shape, and sensitivity) to closely mimic its natural functions; however, its application was limited by a small patient cohort of only 6 individuals, lack of a versatile option for the ideal motion vector, and inability to demonstrate statistical significance in functional outcomes.

Choi and colleagues have significantly contributed to the field categorizing dynamic reconstruction into 3 types based on flap configuration tailored to the defect's requirements,[5,27,59] including the gracilis muscle flap resurfaced with a skin graft, the chimeric ALT flap with vastus lateralis muscle transfer, and the free gracilis flap conjoined with the RFFF (**Fig. 7**). Each approach combines a cutaneous and functional muscle component, with revascularization from the cervical vessels crucial for oral cavity inset.

Choi and colleagues's method addresses the challenges associated with solitary muscle flaps, particularly those without a skin paddle, as such flaps are prone to contraction and may adhere to the surrounding oral mucosa during healing, potentially impairing tongue movement. Incorporating skin paddles was presented as a solution to minimize adhesion and scar contracture, thereby preserving muscle flap mobility. Additionally, they found differences in the anatomic and functional characteristics of the vastus lateralis and gracilis muscles. The vastus lateralis, when used in the chimeric ALT flap, exhibits a variable muscle fiber arrangement dependent on the perforator vessel's location, whereas the gracilis flap provides a consistent muscle fiber arrangement that facilitates more versatile flap insetting.

Despite these anatomic distinctions, they found no significant difference in the functional outcomes among the flap types following dynamic reconstruction, underscoring the effectiveness of these approaches in restoring tongue function.

In Choi's method, the muscle component of the reconstruction is positioned to serve as either a posterolateral vector, emulating the styloglossus muscle's sling motion, or an anteroposterior vector to simulate the hypoglossal sling from the ventrolateral surface[6] (**Fig. 8**). To recreate the styloglossal and/or palatoglossal slings, one end of the transferred muscle is sutured to the palatine aponeurosis or the remaining ends of the styloglossus or palatoglossus muscles; the other end is secured to the residual tongue tissue. Similarly, the hypoglossal sling is reconstructed by attaching one end of the transferred muscle to the soft tissue between the tongue base and hyoid bone, with the opposite end anchored to the residual tongue. Following muscle insertion, the defect's remaining lining is covered with a skin paddle from the flap or a skin graft (**Figs. 9** and **10**).

Functional Outcomes in Dynamic Reconstruction

Electromyographic findings
The restoration of contractile function through neural anastomosis, particularly in preventing muscular atrophy, has been a topic of considerable debate. Several electromyographic studies on reinnervated myocutaneous free flaps reported various outcomes.[40,60,61] Liao and colleagues observed spontaneous actions in the innervated rectus abdominis muscle during swallowing attempts by patients in the follow-up period, suggesting that innervated muscles can regain neural activity in 6 to 12 months postoperatively, supported by standard neurophysiological patterns.[61] Galie and colleagues noted improvements in latency and compound motor action potentials as indicators of effective neural coaptation during follow-ups.[60] Furthermore, the

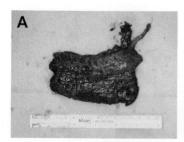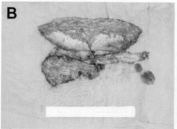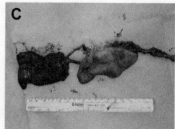

Fig. 7. Various flap configurations for dynamic tongue reconstruction. (*A*) Gracilis muscle free flap, (*B*) chimeric anterolateral thigh flap with vastus lateralis muscle, and (*C*) free gracilis flap conjoined with the RFFF.

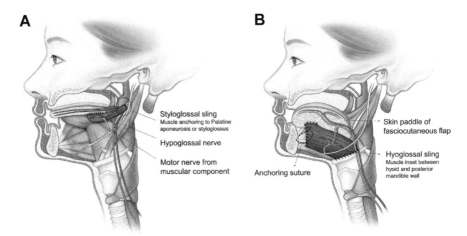

Fig. 8. Schematic illustration of flap inset based on the sling direction. (*A*) While reconstructing the styloglossal and/or palatoglossal sling, surgeons suture one end of the muscle component to either the residual styloglossus muscle or the palatine aponeurosis, while anchoring the other end to the residual tongue tissue. (*B*) For hyoglossal sling reconstruction, one end of the transferred muscle is sutured to the soft tissue between the hyoid bone, and the other end is secured to the posterior mandible wall and remaining tongue tissue. (*From* Refs.[5,6])

effect of postoperative radiation on motor nerve anastomosis has been explored.[62–64] Despite concerns, some studies have reported no negative effect of postoperative radiation on motor nerve reinnervation,[62,63] This suggests that the potential detrimental effects of radiation on neural anastomosis may not be as significant as previously thought, offering promising insights into

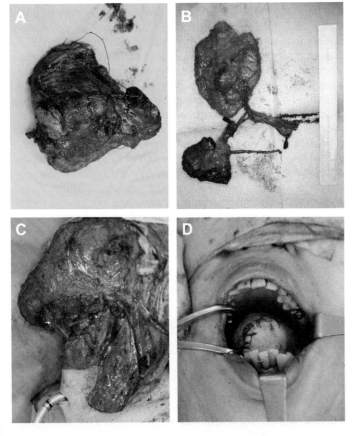

Fig. 9. Subtotal tongue reconstruction with a chimeric ALT and gracilis free flap. (*A*) Tongue and mouth floor specimen after tumor resection. (*B*) Appearance of the chimeric ALT and gracilis free flap. (*C*) The gracilis muscle (*arrow*) positioned in the mouth floor, extending from the posterior of the anterior mandible to the hyoid bone to provide a postero-lateral vector. Note the anastomosis between the obturator nerve and the hypoglossal nerve (*arrowhead*). (*D*) Post-flap inset completion. (*From* Refs.[5,6])

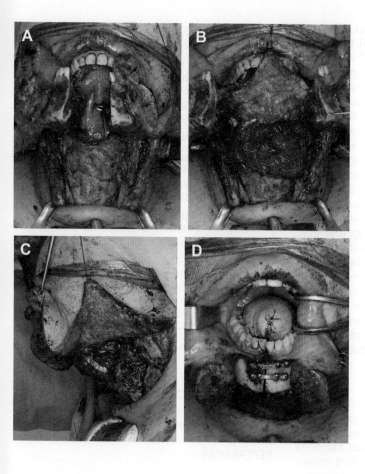

Fig. 10. Total tongue reconstruction using the chimeric ALT and vastus lateralis free flap (*A*) After cancer resection, following total glossectomy. (*B*) The skin paddle from the fasciocutaneous flap shapes the external tongue, with muscle placed in the mouth floor for a hyoglossal sling. (*C*) In the lateral view, the muscle inset shows one end attached to the hyoid bone and the other end secured to the posterior mandibular wall and any remaining tongue tissue. (*D*) The skin paddle is fashioned into a cone shape for the neo-tongue. (*From* Refs.[5,6])

the recovery of nerve function following reconstructive surgery.

Swallowing outcomes

Standardization of swallowing outcomes in reconstructive surgery literature is lacking, making comparisons across studies challenging. Consequently, gastrostomy tube (G-tube) dependency rates were selected as a basic measure for comparison. Systematic reviews revealed that ALT or rectus abdominis flaps are preferred in most reconstructions, avoiding RFFFs due to insufficient tissue volume.[59,65] Choi and colleagues found no significant reduction in G-tube dependency among patients undergoing dynamic reconstruction with chimeric free flaps and innervated muscle flaps.[59] Notably, extensive surgeries, such as bilateral neck dissection and radical or modified radical neck dissection, substantially increased G-tube usage. These findings emphasize that swallowing ability and nutritional support needs are influenced by cancer severity, patients' overall health, and disease progression, rather than just the reconstruction method.

Choi and colleagues conducted a detailed analysis to determine the influence of various factors on VFSS outcomes, adjusting for various confounders[6] and revealed that dynamic reconstruction techniques significantly enhance VFSS scores. After adjusting for multiple variables, the odds ratio for the success of dynamic reconstruction decreased, suggesting its augmented effectiveness, particularly when stratifying patients by the extent of glossectomy or involvement of the tongue base. Hence, Choi and colleagues advocated for the preferential use of dynamic reconstruction in cases involving more than half of the tongue's volume or resection of the tongue base.[6] For surgeries not meeting these criteria, conventional method, aimed at merely filling the surgical void, remains a viable option as it does not contribute to functional decline.

Speech outcomes

Speech outcomes in tongue reconstruction remain a subject of debate within existing research.[6,45,55,57] While motor nerve reinnervation is theorized to prevent the flap tissue atrophy and potentially restore muscles' contractile ability, the ability to enable coordinated, dynamic movements of the flap along with the residual tongue tissue is not conclusively established. Ozkan and colleagues explored the functional reconstruction of total or subtotal glossectomy defects using a chimeric ALT flap with both sensory and motor innervation,[55] with half of the participants demonstrating "good" speech intelligibility and the other half showing "acceptable" outcomes. Righini and colleagues utilized the innervated gracilis musculocutaneous flap following total glossectomy. Their results indicated excellent intelligible speech in 76.9% of the patients and moderately intelligible speech in the remaining 23.1%.[57] However, in contrast, Choi and colleagues's study incorporated a larger cohort of 94 patients and found no significant difference in speech function between patients undergoing dynamic versus conventional reconstruction.[6] This suggests that, while dynamic reconstruction methods show promise in individual cases, the overall advantage of these techniques over traditional methods in improving speech outcomes is not universally established. Future studies should aim to thoroughly document both sensory and motor recovery in free flap reconstructions and assess how these aspects of recovery contribute to improved functional outcomes.

SUMMARY

Successful tongue reconstruction involves multiple factors, including prompt wound healing, careful selection of flaps for improved mobility and volume, and maintaining essential oral functions for optimal rehabilitation outcomes. This review highlights the progress in functional tongue reconstruction, emphasizing key aspects such as flap choice, positioning, volume from a functional perspective, and cutting-edge dynamic reconstruction techniques.

A significant shift toward dynamic reconstruction utilizing motor-innervated free flaps marks a major advancement, aimed at replicating the tongue's natural functions to enhance speech and swallowing significantly. The effectiveness of dynamic methods, evidenced by improvements in swallowing efficiency and speech clarity, highlights their value in facilitating functional tongue rehabilitation.

CLINICS CARE POINTS

Evidence-Based Pearls:

- Flap Choice and Tailoring: Optimal functional tongue reconstruction hinges on selecting the right flap and adjusting its volume and placement meticulously.
- Customized Reconstruction Techniques: Innovations like the perforator flap concept

enable tailored solutions for tongue defects, enhancing anatomic and functional restoration.
- Motor-Innervated Flaps: Utilizing motor-innervated free flaps can significantly improve dynamic tongue reconstruction, enhancing speech and swallowing functions.

Potential Pitfalls:

- Neglecting Flap Design Details: Overlooking the importance of flap shape, inset, and design specificities can compromise the functional replication of the tongue's 3D structure.
- Underestimating Rehabilitation Challenges: Adequate attention is needed for postoperative rehabilitation challenges, especially in dynamic reconstruction methods.
- Inadequate Planning for Radiation Effects: Not accounting for postoperative radiation effects on flap volume can lead to significant volume reduction, impacting functionality.

DISCLOSURE

J.W. Choi and Y.C. Kim have no conflicts of interest, competition of interest, or relevant funding support to disclose in relation to this article.

REFERENCES

1. Urken ML, Moscoso JF, Lawson W, et al. A systematic approach to functional reconstruction of the oral cavity following partial and total glossectomy. Arch Otolaryngol Head Neck Surg 1994; 120(6):589–601.
2. Choi JW, Alshomer F, Kim YC. Current status and evolution of microsurgical tongue reconstructions, part I. Archives of craniofacial surgery 2022;23(4):139–51.
3. Choi JW, Alshomer F, Kim YC. Evolution and current status of microsurgical tongue reconstruction, part II. Archives of craniofacial surgery 2022;23(5):193–204.
4. Park H, Park JS, Jeong WS, et al. Dynamic Hemitongue Defect Reconstruction With Functional Gracilis Muscle Free Transfer. Ann Plast Surg 2021; 86(3):308–16.
5. Kim YC, Woo SH, Jeong WS, et al. Impact of Dynamic Tongue Reconstruction on Sequential Changes of Swallowing Function in Patients Undergoing Total or Near-Total Glossectomy. Ann Plast Surg 2023;91(2):257–64.
6. Choi JW, Kim YC, Park H, et al. The impact of dynamic tongue reconstruction using functional muscle transfer: A retrospective review of 94 cases with functional outcome analysis for various glossectomy defects. Journal of cranio-maxillo-facial surgery 2022;50(9):719–31.

7. Gilbert RW. Reconstruction of the oral cavity; past, present and future. Oral Oncol 2020;108: 104683.

8. Ho AS, Kim S, Tighiouart M, et al. Quantitative survival impact of composite treatment delays in head and neck cancer. Cancer 2018;124(15):3154–62.

9. Chepeha DB, Spector ME, Chinn SB, et al. Hemiglossectomy tongue reconstruction: Modeling of elevation, protrusion, and functional outcome using receiver operator characteristic curve. Head Neck 2016;38(7):1066–73.

10. Matsui Y, Ohno K, Yamashita Y, et al. Factors influencing postoperative speech function of tongue cancer patients following reconstruction with fasciocutaneous/myocutaneous flaps–a multicenter study. Int J Oral Maxillofac Surg 2007;36(7):601–9.

11. Uwiera T, Seikaly H, Rieger J, et al. Functional outcomes after hemiglossectomy and reconstruction with a bilobed radial forearm free flap. J Otolaryngol 2004;33(6):356–9.

12. Vincent A, Kohlert S, Lee TS, et al. Free-Flap Reconstruction of the Tongue. Semin Plast Surg 2019;33(1): 38–45.

13. Ji YB, Cho YH, Song CM, et al. Long-term functional outcomes after resection of tongue cancer: determining the optimal reconstruction method. Eur Arch Oto-Rhino-Laryngol 2017;274(10):3751–6.

14. Bokhari WA, Wang SJ. Tongue reconstruction: recent advances. Curr Opin Otolaryngol Head Neck Surg 2007;15(4):202–7.

15. Ansarin M, Bruschini R, Navach V, et al. Classification of GLOSSECTOMIES: Proposal for tongue cancer resections. Head Neck 2019;41(3):821–7.

16. Bhattacharya S, Thankappan K, Joseph ST, et al. Volume and Location of the Defect as Predictors of Swallowing Outcome After Glossectomy: Correlation with a Classification. Dysphagia 2021;36(6):974–83.

17. Mannelli G, Arcuri F, Agostini T, et al. Classification of tongue cancer resection and treatment algorithm. J Surg Oncol 2018;117(5):1092–9.

18. Butler DP, Dunne JA, Wood SH, et al. A Unifying Algorithm in Microvascular Reconstruction of Oral Cavity Defects Using the Trilaminar Concept. Plastic and reconstructive surgery Global open 2019;7(7): e2267.

19. Liu WW, Zhang CY, Li JY, et al. A novel classification system for the evaluation and reconstruction of oral defects following oncological surgery. Oncol Lett 2017;14(6):7049–54.

20. Hanasono MM, Matros E, Disa JJ. Important aspects of head and neck reconstruction. Plast Reconstr Surg 2014;134(6):968e–80e.

21. Kimata Y, Sakuraba M, Hishinuma S, et al. Analysis of the relations between the shape of the reconstructed tongue and postoperative functions after subtotal or total glossectomy. Laryngoscope 2003; 113(5):905–9.

22. Yun IS, Lee DW, Lee WJ, et al. Correlation of neo-tongue volume changes with functional outcomes after long-term follow-up of total glossectomy. J Craniofac Surg 2010;21(1):111–6.

23. Jeong HH, Jeong WS, Choi JW, et al. 3D computer simulation analysis of the flap volume change in total tongue reconstruction flaps. Journal of cranio-maxillo-facial surgery 2018;46(5):844–50.

24. Cho KJ, Joo YH, Sun DI, et al. Perioperative clinical factors affecting volume changes of reconstructed flaps in head and neck cancer patients: free versus regional flaps. Eur Arch Oto-Rhino-Laryngol 2011; 268(7):1061–5.

25. Tarsitano A, Battaglia S, Cipriani R, et al. Microvascular reconstruction of the tongue using a free anterolateral thigh flap: Three-dimensional evaluation of volume loss after radiotherapy. Journal of cranio-maxillo-facial surgery 2016;44(9):1287–91.

26. Bittermann G, Thönissen P, Poxleitner P, et al. Microvascular transplants in head and neck reconstruction: 3D evaluation of volume loss. Journal of cranio-maxillo-facial surgery 2015;43(8):1319–24.

27. Woo SH, Kim YC, Jeong WS, et al. Three-Dimensional Analysis of Flap Volume Change in Total Tongue Reconstruction: Focus on Reinnervated Dynamic Tongue Reconstruction. J Craniofac Surg 2023;34(7):2056–60.

28. Hsiao HT, Leu YS, Lin CC. Tongue reconstruction with free radial forearm flap after hemiglossectomy: a functional assessment. J Reconstr Microsurg 2003;19(3):137–42.

29. Davison SP, Grant NN, Schwarz KA, et al. Maximizing flap inset for tongue reconstruction. Plast Reconstr Surg 2008;121(6):1982–5.

30. Chiu T, Burd A. Our technique of "tongue" folding. Plast Reconstr Surg 2009;123(1):426–7.

31. Chepeha DB, Teknos TN, Shargorodsky J, et al. Rectangle tongue template for reconstruction of the hemiglossectomy defect. Arch Otolaryngol Head Neck Surg 2008;134(9):993–8.

32. Choi JW, Lee MY, Oh TS. The application of multilobed flap designs for anatomic and functional oropharyngeal reconstructions. J Craniofac Surg 2013;24(6):2091–7.

33. Seikaly H, Rieger J, O'Connell D, et al. Beavertail modification of the radial forearm free flap in base of tongue reconstruction: technique and functional outcomes. Head Neck 2009;31(2):213–9.

34. Dziegielewski PT, Rieger J, Shama MA, et al. Beavertail modification of the radial forearm free flap in total oral glossectomy reconstruction: Technique and functional outcomes. Oral Oncol 2019;96: 71–6.

35. Longo B, Pagnoni M, Ferri G, et al. The mushroom-shaped anterolateral thigh perforator flap for subtotal tongue reconstruction. Plast Reconstr Surg 2013; 132(3):656–65.

36. Zhou X, He ZJ, Su YX, et al. "Sushi roll" technique for precise total tongue functional reconstruction using a pre-sutured femoral anterolateral myocutaneous flap. Oral Oncol 2020;110:104866.

37. Sakuraba M, Asano T, Miyamoto S, et al. A new flap design for tongue reconstruction after total or subtotal glossectomy in thin patients. J Plast Reconstr Aesthetic Surg : JPRAS 2009;62(6):795–9.

38. Koumoullis H, Burley O, Kyzas P. Patient-specific soft tissue reconstruction: an IDEAL stage I report of hemiglossectomy reconstruction and introduction of the PANSOFOS flap. Br J Oral Maxillofac Surg 2020;58(6):681–6.

39. Stone M, Woo J, Lee J, et al. Structure and variability in human tongue muscle anatomy. Computer methods in biomechanics and biomedical engineering Imaging & visualization 2018;6(5):499–507.

40. Yamamoto Y, Sugihara T, Furuta Y, et al. Functional reconstruction of the tongue and deglutition muscles following extensive resection of tongue cancer. Plast Reconstr Surg 1998;102(4):993–8 [discussion: 999–1000].

41. Manrique OJ, Leland HA, Langevin CJ, et al. Optimizing Outcomes following Total and Subtotal Tongue Reconstruction: A Systematic Review of the Contemporary Literature. J Reconstr Microsurg 2017;33(2):103–11.

42. Kim YC, Lee SJ, Park H, et al. Swallowing analysis in hemi-tongue reconstruction using motor-innervated free flaps: A cine-magnetic resonance imaging study. Head Neck 2023;45(5):1097–112.

43. Matsui Y, Shirota T, Yamashita Y, et al. Analyses of speech intelligibility in patients after glossectomy and reconstruction with fasciocutaneous/myocutaneous flaps. Int J Oral Maxillofac Surg 2009;38(4):339–45.

44. Sun J, Weng Y, Li J, et al. Analysis of determinants on speech function after glossectomy. Journal of oral and maxillofacial surgery 2007;65(10):1944–50.

45. Lam L, Samman N. Speech and swallowing following tongue cancer surgery and free flap reconstruction–a systematic review. Oral Oncol 2013;49(6):507–24.

46. Shin YS, Koh YW, Kim SH, et al. Radiotherapy deteriorates postoperative functional outcome after partial glossectomy with free flap reconstruction. Journal of oral and maxillofacial surgery 2012;70(1):216–20.

47. Yi CR, Jeong WS, Oh TS, et al. Analysis of Speech and Functional Outcomes in Tongue Reconstruction after Hemiglossectomy. J Reconstr Microsurg 2020;36(7):507–13.

48. Ravindra A, Nayak DR, Devaraja K, et al. Functional Outcomes After Surgical Resection of Tongue Cancer; A Comparative Study Between Primary Closure, Secondary Intention Healing and Flap Reconstruction. Indian journal of otolaryngology and head and neck surgery 2022;74(Suppl 3):6296–306.

49. Rui X, Huang Z, Zuo J, et al. Application of an L-shaped anterolateral thigh flap in reconstruction after hemiglossectomy. BMC Surg 2022;22(1):32.

50. Fan S, Li QX, Zhang HQ, et al. "Five-point eight-line" anatomic flap design for precise hemitongue reconstruction. Head Neck 2019;41(5):1359–66.

51. Fujimoto Y, Matsuura H, Kawabata K, et al. [Assessment of Swallowing Ability Scale for oral and oropharyngeal cancer patients]. Nihon Jibiinkoka Gakkai kaiho 1997;100(11):1401–7.

52. Pedersen A, Wilson J, McColl E, et al. Swallowing outcome measures in head and neck cancer–How do they compare? Oral Oncol 2016;52:104–8.

53. Thankappan K, Kuriakose MA, Chatni SS, et al. Lateral arm free flap for oral tongue reconstruction: an analysis of surgical details, morbidity, and functional and aesthetic outcome. Ann Plast Surg 2011;66(3):261–6.

54. Yoleri L, Mavioğlu H. Total tongue reconstruction with free functional gracilis muscle transplantation: a technical note and review of the literature. Ann Plast Surg 2000;45(2):181–6.

55. Ozkan O, Ozkan O, Derin AT, et al. True functional reconstruction of total or subtotal glossectomy defects using a chimeric anterolateral thigh flap with both sensorial and motor innervation. Ann Plast Surg 2015;74(5):557–64.

56. Sharma M, Iyer S, Kuriakose MA, et al. Functional reconstruction of near total glossectomy defects using composite gastro omental-dynamic gracilis flaps. J Plast Reconstr Aesthetic Surg : JPRAS 2009;62(10):1277–80.

57. Righini S, Festa BM, Bonanno MC, et al. Dynamic tongue reconstruction with innervated gracilis musculocutaneos flap after total glossectomy. Laryngoscope 2019;129(1):76–81.

58. Calabrese L, Saito A, Navach V, et al. Tongue reconstruction with the gracilis myocutaneous free flap. Microsurgery 2011;31(5):355–9.

59. Stewart T, Copeland-Halperin LR, Demsas F, et al. Predictors of gastrostomy tube placement in patients with head and neck cancer undergoing resection and flap-based reconstruction: systematic review and meta-analysis. J Plast Reconstr Aesthetic Surg : JPRAS 2023;79:1–10.

60. Galiè E, Villani V, Ferreli F, et al. Vastus lateralis myofascial free flap for tongue reconstruction and hypoglossal-femoral anastomosis: neurophysiological study. Neurol Sci 2019;40(3):553–9.

61. Liao G, Su Y, Zhang J, et al. Reconstruction of the tongue with reinnervated rectus abdominis musculoperitoneal flaps after hemiglossectomy. J Laryngol Otol 2006;120(3):205–13.

62. Gidley PW, Herrera SJ, Hanasono MM, et al. The impact of radiotherapy on facial nerve repair. Laryngoscope 2010;120(10):1985–9.

63. Yi CR, Oh TM, Jeong WS, et al. Quantitative analysis of the impact of radiotherapy on facial nerve repair with sural nerve grafting after parotid gland surgery. Journal of cranio-maxillo-facial surgery 2020;48(8):724–32.

64. Hontanilla B, Qiu SS, Marré D. Effect of postoperative brachytherapy and external beam radiotherapy on functional outcomes of immediate facial nerve repair after radical parotidectomy. Head Neck 2014;36(1):113–9.

65. Rieger JM, Tang JA, Harris J, et al. Survey of current functional outcomes assessment practices in patients with head and neck cancer: initial project of the head and neck research network. J Otolaryngol Head Neck Surg 2010;39(5):523–31.

The Anterolateral Thigh Flap in Head and Neck Reconstruction

Jingya Jane Pu, BDS, MDS[a], Andrew Atia, MD[b], Peirong Yu, MD, MS[b], Yu-Xiong Su, MD, PhD[a],*

KEYWORDS

- Head and neck reconstruction • Anterolateral thigh flap • Free flap • Microsurgery • Oral cancer
- Surgical planning

KEY POINTS

- Anterolateral thigh (ALT) flap is one of the most important workhorse flaps in head and neck reconstruction.
- It can be harvested either as a fasciocutaneous flap or a musculocutaneous flap with the inclusion of vastus lateralis (VL) muscle for defects of different sizes.
- The motor nerve to VL can be harvested together with the muscle to provide function of the muscle for oral tongue reconstruction.
- The anteromedial thigh flap based on the perforators from the rectus femoris branch can be harvested as a backup when the perforator for the ALT is absent or as a chimeric flap with the ALT for reconstruction of complex head and neck defects.

INTRODUCTION
Background

The anterolateral thigh (ALT) flap was first described by Song and colleagues in 1984[1] and popularized for its application in head and neck reconstruction by Koshima and colleagues in 1993.[2] Since then, it has become a popular choice among surgeons worldwide.

The ALT flap is a versatile flap that can be used for various indications, such as oral cavity reconstruction, pharyngeal and esophageal repair, skin resurfacing, and skull base reconstruction. The flap can be harvested as a free fascia or fasciocutaneous flap with variable amount of skin, fascia and fat, or as as a free myocutaneous flap with a cuff of vastus lateralis (VL) muscle, tensor fasciae latae (TFL) muscle, or both, allowing the chimeric design for the reconstruction of complex defects of head and neck at a single stage.

The ALT flap is based on perforators from the descending branch of the lateral circumflex femoral artery (LCFA), which provides a long and sizable vascular pedicle. Its location away from the head allows comfortable simultaneous 2 team approach for head and neck reconstruction. The donor site morbidity is minimal, as the thigh defect can be closed primarily or with a split-thickness skin graft, leaving a well-concealed scar, and minimal impact on the function of the thigh in the long-term.

[a] Division of Oral and Maxillofacial Surgery, Faculty of Dentistry, The University of Hong Kong, Prince Philip Dental Hospital, 34 Hospital Road, Sai Ying Pun, Hong Kong; [b] Department of Plastic Surgery, The University of Texas MD Anderson Cancer Center, Houston, TX, USA
* Corresponding author.
E-mail address: richsu@hku.hk

Oral Maxillofacial Surg Clin N Am 36 (2024) 451–462
https://doi.org/10.1016/j.coms.2024.07.001
1042-3699/24/© 2024 Elsevier Inc. All rights are reserved, including those for text and data mining, AI training, and similar technologies.

However, concerns also exist for ALT flap due to the variability of its vascular anatomy and perforator location, the potential for partial flap necrosis, and the large variation in flap thickness in different populations. The success of the ALT flap depends on careful preoperative planning, meticulous flap harvest, proper flap inset, and post-operative care.

This review aims to provide a comprehensive overview of the ALT flap, including its surgical anatomy, step-by-step surgical technique, clinical applications, anatomic variations, complications, and management strategies.

SURGICAL ANATOMY OF THE ANTEROLATERAL THIGH FLAP
Anatomic Landmarks

The main anatomic landmarks for ALT flap harvest include anterior superior iliac spine (ASIS), lateral point of patella, and femoral artery identified by the palpation of its pulse (**Fig. 1**A, B).

Vascular Supply of the Anterolateral Thigh Flap

The ALT flap is supplied predominantly by the descending branch and alternatively by the transverse or oblique branch of the LCFA. LCFA arises from the lateral side of the profunda femoris, passes horizontally behind the rectus femoris (RF) muscle, and gives off the branches. Either the branches or the LCFA itself can be harvested as vascular pedicle for microvascular anastomosis.

Perforator Anatomy

Almost all (98.6%) of the patients have at least 1 cutaneous perforator. The number of perforators range from 1 to 3 with an average count of 2.04. Most of the perforators have some intramuscular course in the VL. The perforators of the ALT flap typically arise from the descending branch of the LCFA in 90% of the patients and can be identified along a line drawn from the ASIS and

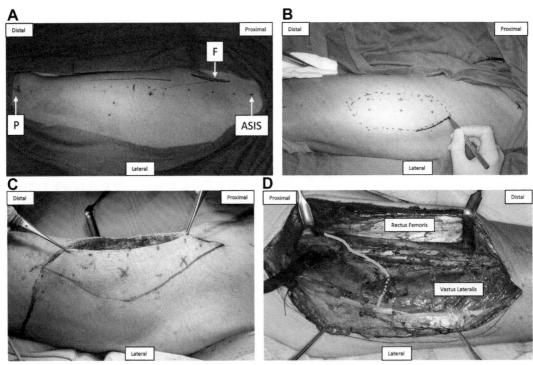

Fig. 1. Design of anterolateral thigh (ALT) free flap. (*A*) Anatomic landmarks. Anterior Superior Iliac Spine (ASIS). Lateral point of patella (P). Femoral artery (F). The rough location of the septum between the rectus femoris and the vastus lateralis is marked by a line connecting the ASIS and the lateral patella (AP line). (*B*) The flap is outlined on the axis of the septum dividing the vastus lateralis and the rectus femoris muscles, centered at the midpoint between ASIS and P or on the preoperatively identified perforators. (*C*) Incision made medial to the axis of a line from the ASIS to the superior central aspect of the patella can be used to capture perforators to the ALT flap and adapted when necessary for harvest of the anteromedial thigh (AMT) flap or TFL perforator flap when ALT perforators are anatomically absent or insufficient (*D*) The course of the perforator is marked in green. The dotted line indicates the muscular course of perforator in the vastus lateralis. Careful dissection is required to fully reveal the course before ligation of the pedicle.

superior lateral patella (AP line).[3] (**Fig. 1**) The most common location of the perforator is at the midpoint of the AP line, with the other 2 possible perforators located within 5 cm away from it. In horizontal dimension, perforators are on average found 1.4 cm lateral to the AP line, so an incision made medial to the axis of a line from the ASIS to the superior central aspect of the patella can be used to capture perforators to the ALT flap and adapted when necessary for harvest of the anteromedial thigh (AMT) flap or TFL perforator flap when ALT perforators are anatomically absent or insufficient. The anatomic variations and management strategies will be discussed in the later section.

Innervation

The sensation of ALT flap skin paddle comes from the lateral femoral cutaneous nerve. It can be harvested together with the flap to provide sensation for the tongue and oropharynx (**Fig. 2**).[4] When muscle function is desired, VL muscle can be harvested together with its motor branches from the posterior division of femoral nerve accompanying the descending branch of the LFCA.

STEP-BY-STEP SURGICAL PROCEDURE

1. *Patient selection and preoperative planning*: Preoperative assessment of both the donor site and the recipient defect is crucial for selecting the appropriate flap. The thickness of the ALT flap varies significantly among individuals. When the thickness of the ALT is less than ideal, other flap choices should be considered. When tissue at the thigh is too thin, profunda artery perforator, latissimus dorsi, or rectus abdominis free flaps can be considered as alternatives. However, ALT is often thicker than what is required. In such cases, super-thin ALT, lateral arm, or radial forearm flap should be harvested instead. The comparisons of different flaps are shown in **Table 1**.

2. *Patient positioning*: The patient is placed in a supine position. The ALT can be comfortably accessed with the operator sitting on the lateral side of the thigh and 1 assistant sitting on each side of the table.

3. *Donor site marking and flap design*: After standard disinfection and draping, the anatomic landmarks are drawn. Location of skin perforators can be detected traditionally by doppler. Machine requirement and techniques have

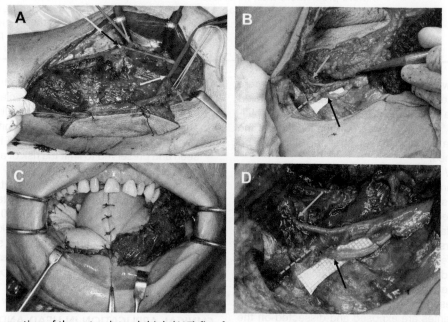

Fig. 2. Innervation of the anterolateral thigh (ALT) flap for tongue reconstruction after subtotal glossectomy. (*A*) The anatomy before division of vascular pedicle. Green arrow: descending branch of lateral circumflex femoral artery (LCFA). Black arrow: motor nerve to vastus lateralis. Yellow arrow: branch of LCFA to tensor fascia Lata. Blue arrow: lateral femoral cutaneous nerve. (*B*) After inset of flap and anastomosis. Green arrow: arterial anastomosis to facial artery. Green dotted arrow: venous anastomosis with venous coupler to a branch of common facial vein. Black arrow: anastomosis of motor nerve to vastus lateralis with proximal end of hypoglossal nerve. Motor nerve to vastus lateralis anastomosed with proximal end of hypoglossal nerve. (*C*) After flap inset. (*D*) Close-up view of the neurovascular anastomosis.

Table 1
The alternative choices with their advantages and disadvantages compared

Flap Type	Advantages	Disadvantages
Lateral arm flap	• Hidden linear scar at the upper arm • Pliable tissue • Reliable septocutaneous perforators • Satisfactory length of pedicle	• Donor site close to head and neck resection site, crowded. • Vessel caliber might be small and dissection into the spiral groove is required for better vessel size
Rectus Abdominis Free Flap	• Can be harvested without changing patient position. • Substantial volume. • Sufficiently long pedicle of epigastric artery.	• Risk of hernia • Muscle atrophy at recipient site in long term • Significant postoperative pain • Variation in harvested volume due to big variation of adipose tissue thickness
Latissimus Dorsi Free Flap	• Abundant volume of tissue and good pedicle length. • Minimal donor site morbidity and hidden scar with clothing.	• Difficult simultaneous two-team approach for head and neck reconstruction. • Muscle atrophy at recipient site in long term.
Profunda Artery Perforator Flap	• Hidden scar • Can be harvested with innervated gracilis muscle to provide both isotonic and isometric contractions facilitating both larynx and tongue elevation in patients after glossectomy.[7] The movement is more predictable than innervated vastus lateralis with ALT flap.	• An adequate vascular configuration to harvest the chimeric flap is present in <30% of the population.[8] • CTA and duplex ultrasound are required to identify patients who are candidates for reconstruction with a chimeric PAP–gracilis flap. • False positives could appear and the joining of the two pedicles may not be found during the surgical procedure. Two independent pairs of anastomoses may be required.

been well described.[5] Recently, thermocamera attached to the smart phone has been proved to be a reliable technique for perforator identification.[6–8] (**Fig. 3**) Based on the location of the perforators and defect size, the flap can be designed.

4. *Medial incision and flap elevation*: The medial incision is made through skin and subcutaneous tissue down to fascia lata. The flap is elevated from the RF muscle laterally either suprafascial or subfascial dissection. The perforators are identified and preserved.

5. *Pedicle identification*: The septum between the RF and the VL muscle is identified. With the 2 muscles easily separated with digit dissection, the descending branch of LCFA and its venae comitantes are exposed and dissected off the fascia (**Fig. 1**D).

6. *Perforator dissection*: The courses of the perforating vessels are revealed by retrograde dissection from the skin perforators and antegrade dissection from the pedicle.

7. *Flap harvest*: Lateral incision is then made with the desired width and length of the skin paddle

after confirming the defect size with the tumor resection team. A cuff of VL muscle can be included based on the defect requirements. The pedicle is dissected toward its bifurcation from the LCFA. A sizable branch to RF is usually seen and preserved to limit the risk of avascular necrosis of the RF muscle.

8. *Closure and postoperative care*: A suction drain is inserted after meticulous hemostasis and kept until the output is less than 20 mL per 24 hours. The wound can usually be closed primarily with a linear scar. When a small skin graft is required, it can be easily be harvested from the thigh along the proximal incision where the tension is minimal.

CLINICAL APPLICATION IN HEAD AND NECK RECONSTRUCTION

Due to its versatility, ALT flap has been used for reconstruction of different kinds of soft tissue defects in head and neck. We review a couple of common clinical reconstruction scenarios as follows.

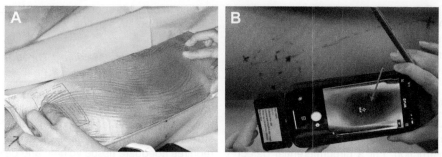

Fig. 3. Thermocamera for skin perforator (*red arrow* in *B*) identification. (*A*) Cold challenge with gel pad. (*B*) The area supplied by the perforator will warm up faster than the other parts of the skin thus shown as a light spot on the thermocamera.

Reconstruction for Glossectomy Defects

For subtotal and total glossectomy defects, the tissue bulk measured in its vertical dimension is the key for satisfactory swallowing function (**Fig. 4**).[9] The dorsum of the neotongue should be able to touch the palate during swallowing to push food to the hypopharynx and deliver food to the lateral gutters to minimize aspiration. ALT musculocutaneous flap provides the required tissue bulk by the inclusion of VL muscle. Provided with good seal at the floor of mouth to isolate oral cavity from the neck, muscle and subcutaneous fat can be exposed to the oral cavity to allow "mucosalization". The motor branch to VL muscle can be anastomosed to the hypoglossal nerve for a functional reconstruction but the improvement in functional and quality of life are yet to be proved

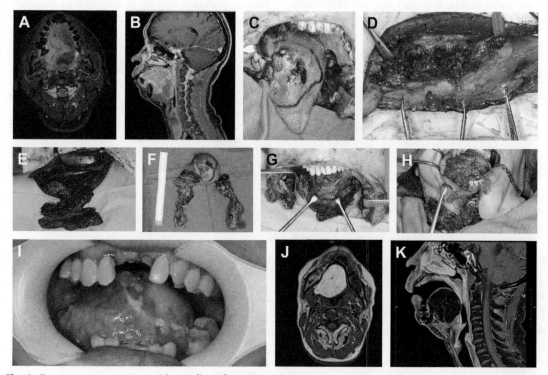

Fig. 4. Tongue reconstruction with ALT flap after subtotal glossectomy for oral squamous cell carcinoma. (*A*) MRI showing the extension of tumor at right tongue crossing midline (axial view) (*B*) Sagittal view. (*C*) Tumor identified clinically. (*D*) Dissection of vastus lateralis to expose the course of musculocutaneous perforators. (*E*) Flap harvested with a cuff of vastus lateralis muscle. (*F*) Subtotal glossectomy with bilateral neck dissection specimen. (*G*) Remaining defect. (*H*) After inset of ALT with exposed fat and muscle to the oral cavity. (*I*) Early postoperative appearance. (*J*) MRI showing the reconstructed tongue at postoperative 2 years (Axial view). (*K*) Sagittal view. Note the relationship of neotongue with the palate. Good swallowing function was achieved.

(see **Fig. 2**). For a smaller defect after partial glossectomy, ALT is a less common choice than radial forearm and lateral arm flaps. However, this also depends on the size match of the estimated volume of the defect and the thickness of the ALT flap.

Reconstruction for Pharyngoesophageal Defects

ALT flap is also widely used for pharyngoesophageal reconstruction. For a circumferential defect after total laryngectomy, a flap of 9 cm wide is typically harvested (**Fig. 5**). When 2 or more cutaneous perforators are identified, separate skin islands can be used for pharyngoesophageal reconstruction and anterior neck resurfacing at the same time (see **Fig. 5**). If not possible, various amount of VL muscle can be easily harvested based on the same vascular pedicle for neck resurfacing and tracheostoma reconstruction. ALT flaps showed higher success rate for speech rehabilitation with tracheoesophageal puncture prosthesis, better spontaneous swallowing performance, and shorter hospital stays than jejunal flaps. The rate of fistula formation is also lower. It might be due to the extra fascia that can be harvested with ALT flaps which provides an extra layer of suturing leading to possible spontaneous healing of fistulas in the postoperative period.[10]

Reconstruction for Maxillary Through-and-Through Defect

A maxilla through-and-through defect involves the loss of the palate, the upper alveolar ridge, the nasal floor and the facial skin (**Fig. 6**). The reconstruction of this complex three-dimensional defect requires adequate tissue volume and delicate flap inset to restore the functions of speech, swallowing, the facial appearance. An ALT flap can be used to reconstruct this defect with a single-stage procedure. The flap is de-epithelialized at the superior end and rotated inward, together with the VL muscle, they increase the tissue bulk and support for the midface for a better facial contour. To repair the surface defects at both facial skin and oral cavity, the skin paddle is de-epithelialized in the middle to create a buried segment, which will be connected to the inner surface of the upper lip after healing. Depending on the choice of recipient vessels, tunneling to the neck or preauricular area is usually required. Nasopharyngeal airway is inserted to maintain the space of nasal cavity during healing. The flap

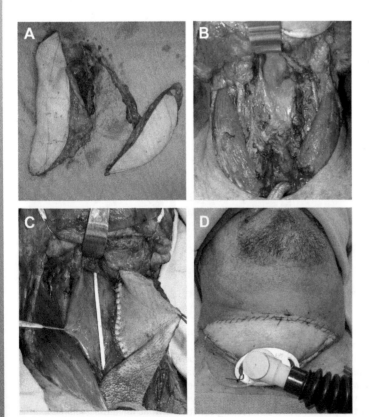

Fig. 5. Reconstruction for the pharyngoesophageal defect with the chimeric anterolateral thigh-anteromedial thigh (ALT-AMT) flap. (*A*) ALT + AMT. (*B*) Defect. (*C*) Reconstruction. (*D*) Resurfacing.

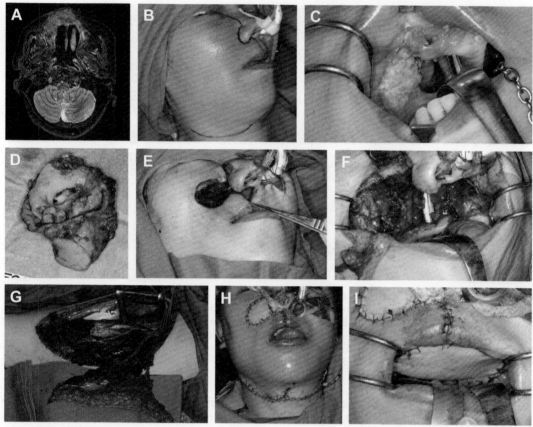

Fig. 6. Maxilla through-and-through defect reconstruction with anterolateral thigh (ALT). (*A*) MRI showing squamous cell carcinoma (SCC) at maxillary gingiva with proximity to skin surface. (*B*) Skin erythema observed indicating possible tumor invasion. (*C*) Tumor exposed intraorally. (*D*) Tumor resected. (*E*) Residual extraoral defect. (*F*) Residual intraoral defect with communication to maxillary sinus and nasal cavity. (*G*) ALT flap harvested with a cuff of vastus lateralis muscle. (*H*) After reconstruction (extraoral view). (*I*) Intraoral view.

is sutured to the remaining palatal mucosa, the nasal mucosa, and the skin margins.

Skull Base Reconstruction

The defect after tumor resection involving the skull base has posed a special challenge for the reconstructive surgeons (**Fig. 7**). Traditionally, local or regional flaps, such as the pericranial flap or temporalis flap are used. However, these options often fail to provide sufficient seal and support for extensive defects, particularly troubling if postoperative radiation therapy is indicated. There are also concerns about blood supply at the distal portion of the local flap leading to partial necrosis and wound dehiscence.

ALT flap has gained popularity over the years for skull base reconstruction due to several advantages. ALT can effectively reconstruct the defects at the intracranial space, cranial base and the infratemporal fossa. It provides enough tissue bulk to support neural and vascular structures.

Its reliable blood supply ensures optimal wound healing. The watertight dural seal provided by ALT prevents cerebrospinal fluid leaks, ascending infections, and pneumocephalus.

Superficial temporal artery and vein are the most used recipient vessels due to its proximity and good match of caliber. When coronal flap is required, preserving the vessels is critical. If the vessels are accidently damaged, retrograde tracing into the parotid can be attempted. If not possible, alternative options will be the vessels from the neck (such as the facial artery) or contralateral vessels, although a longer donor pedicle is necessary, which is usually not a problem for ALT flaps.

As muscles shrink in the postoperative period, surgeons should harvest as much subcutaneous fat and fascia as possible to maintain a stable tissue bulk. The excess tissue can be easily trimmed during inset. Depending on the structure of the defect, thorough de-epithelialization is performed while keeping the dermal plexus intact. The de-epithelialized surface is usually used for the cranial fossa, while the

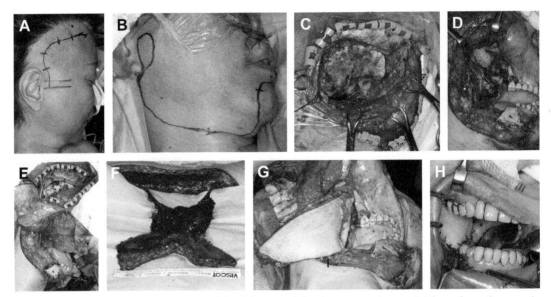

Fig. 7. Post-radiation sarcoma at right condyle. (*A*) Coronal flap to expose the cranial fossa from the superior, taking care not to injure superficial temporal vessels when elevating the flap. (*B*) Skin incision for exposing the tumor from lateral and inferior. (*C*) Brain retracted superiorly to expose the cranial fossa. Cranial base next to the tumor was removed. (*D*) Defect after the segmental mandibulectomy (inferior view). (*E*) Lateral view. (*F*) ALT flap with a cuff of vastus lateralis muscle. (*G*) Flap inset. Note the de-epithelialized subcutaneous tissue for the skull base and inner side of the lip. (*H*) After closure of the intraoral defect and insertion of the guide flange prosthesis.

skin surface is utilized for the lining of maxillary sinus and oral cavity. Postoperative care includes using a suction drain, monitoring in the intensive care unit dedicated for neurosurgical patients, and maintaining head elevation to prevent retrograde flow of wound discharge into the cranial fossa.

Double Free Flaps for Both Soft and Hard Tissues Defects

For large tumors from the mandible with invasion of facial skin, the resection often results in composite defects at the jaw, oral mucosa, and facial skin (**Fig. 8**). Fibula offers an excellent choice for the reconstruction of mandible and intraoral mucosal defect.[11] However, the extraoral skin defect often requires some extra amount of vascularized soft tissue for wound healing and plate coverage to avoid plate exposure after postoperative radiotherapy. ALT with its proficient subcutaneous adipose tissue and fascia often offers a perfect option. Its long pedicle length also provides more versatility in vessel depleted neck if contralateral or more distantly located recipient vessels are desired.

ANATOMIC VARIATIONS AND MANAGEMENT STRATEGIES

Although most patients have consistent anatomy as described in the previous sections, variations do exist. Understanding these variations and their

management strategies is crucial for predictable surgical results. (1) The presence of perforators varies. Careful anatomic study of the perforator pattern in ALT flaps demonstrates that the most commonly available perforator is the perforator located near the midpoint of the line drawn from the ASIS and the superior lateral patella (AP line), which is present in 87% of thighs.[3] The perforator located 5 cm proximal to the midpoint is present in 53%, and the perforator located 5 cm distal to the midpoint, in 59% of thighs. Half of the patients had 2 perforators, a quarter of patients had 1 perforator, and the other quarter of patients had 3 perforators. (2) The size of perforators varies. Proximal perforators tend to be larger than distal perforators. Proximal perforators are also more likely to be septocutaneous ones whereas distal perforators tend to be more musculocutaneous. (3) The origin of perforators varies. In the majority of cases (96%), the perforators originate from the descending branch (Type I origin). In 2% of the cases; however, the perforator may arise from the transverse branch of the LCFA (type II origin). In these cases, the perforator usually travels within the VL muscle for its entire length requiring tedious intramuscular dissection. In another 2% of the cases, the perforator may be encountered above the deep fascia through the initial anterior incision and pierces the RF muscle medial to the septum. By tracing this perforator through the RF muscle, its origin can

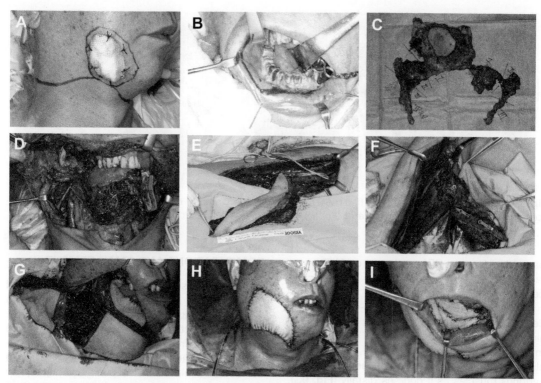

Fig. 8. Squamous cell carcinoma (SCC) at mandible gingiva resected and reconstructed with ALT and fibula free flaps. (*A*) Extraoral incision. (*B*) Intraoral incision. (*C*) Segmental mandibulectomy with bilateral neck dissection specimen. (*D*) Residual defect. (*E*) ALT harvested with a cuff of vastus lateralis muscle. (*F*) Three segment fibula free flap fixed with 3D-printed patient-specific Ti plates. (*G*) Skin paddle of ALT was split into two based on two individual perforators. (*H*) Inferior hal half of the ALT was used to close the skin defect. (*I*) The superior half was rotated intraorally to close the mucosal defect together with the skin paddle of fibula free flap.

be found in the RF vascular branch traveling along the medial edge of the RF muscle. This type III origin was later confirmed as the anteromedial thigh flap perforator. Once this perforator is encountered in the beginning of flap dissection, the surgeon must explore the ALT flap territory more laterally to look for true ALT perforators, which are always lateral to or through the septum between the RF and VL muscles, before dividing this perforator. (4) Perforators can be absent or too small to be clinical useful. In our study, we found that 4.3% of thighs had no suitable perforators in the ALT flap territory. We explored the contralateral thighs in these cases and found that one-third of these had no suitable ALT perforators on the contralateral thigh either (1.4% overall).[12] Unsuccessful exploration of the contralateral thigh results in wasted time, additional incisions, and the potential for increased operative morbidity. In addition, approximately one-quarter of the ALT flaps only had 1 cutaneous perforator. The single perforator anatomy can become problematic when 2 skin paddles are required. In these unfavorable scenarios, the AMT flap may become a rescue.

ANTEROMEDIAL THIGH FLAP

In early publications, the vascular supply of the AMT flap was described as an innominate branch of the LCFA. Confusions arose when more medial perforators were found to originate from the superficial femoral artery (SFA). This configuration; however, is often less favorable due to shorter pedicle length and smaller vessel caliber. In order to clarify the vascular anatomy of the AMT flap, a prospective study was conducted to map the ALT and AMT perforators through the same incision (**Fig. 9**A). In our prospective study, we have found that there are 2 sources of blood supply to the AMT flap. In most cases the AMT flap is perfused by the RF branch, which originates from the proximal part of the descending branch of the LCFA. This is the dominant blood supply to the AMT flap. The other source of blood supply comes from direct small branches from the SFA deep to the vastus intermedius muscle. They are never found coursing through the RF muscle. These SFA perforators are less useful clinically because they are small and short. We, thus, consider the

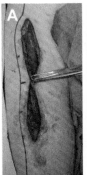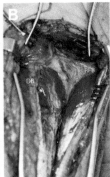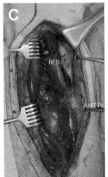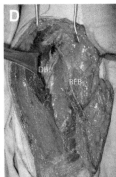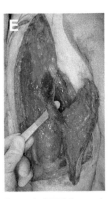

Fig. 9. Harvest of anteromedial thigh flap (AMT). (*A*) Incision. (*B*) Origin of rectus femoris branch (RFB) from descending branch (DB). (*C*) AMT perforator (Pr.) (*D*) AMT flap. (*E*) AMT pedicle.

perforators from the RF branch are true AMT perforators and the RF branch is the true vascular pedicle of the AMT flap.

The RF branch after its take-off from the descending branch travels medially on the underside of the muscle (**Fig. 9**B), then passes in the muscular triangle formed by the RF, vastus medialis and sartorius to finally lie between the RF and sartorius muscles as it courses distally (**Fig. 9**C). The perforators from the RF branch never travel through the sartorius muscle. This is a clear distinction from the SFA perforators.

The majority of AMT perforators are concentrated near the midpoint (point 0.5) of the line connecting the ASIS with the superolateral corner of the patella (AP line), similar to ALT perforators. A long (7–15 cm) and sizable vascular pedicle similar to the ALT flap can usually be generated for the AMT flap (see **Fig. 8**D, E). Most commonly (66% of cases), perforators are septocutaneous while the remaining perforators traverse a short segment of RF muscle.

One important finding from our study is that only 51% of the thighs had AMT perforator(s). Therefore, the value of the AMT flap is to serve as a "back-up" flap when unfavorable perforator anatomy is encountered during ALT flap dissection. We found a reciprocal relationship between ALT and AMT perforators. There is an increased likelihood of AMT perforators being present when ALT perforators are anatomically absent.[12–14] If only 1 ALT perforator is identified, an AMT perforator can be found in approximately 75% of cases. Given the inverse relationship between ALT and AMT perforators, a concept known as reciprocal dominance, care should be maintained to avoid injury to medial perforators upon initial exploration for ALT perforators. Therefore, the AMT flap is an excellent alternative flap option when ALT perforators are absent.

COMPLICATIONS AND MANAGEMENT

The ALT flap is a highly reliable flap option and considered by reconstructive surgeons to be a "workhorse" flap in head and neck reconstruction. In a retrospective review of 3090 consecutive head and neck free flap reconstructions, 40 flap losses occurred, and an overall flap success rate of 98.7% was achieved.[15] In experienced hands, flap success exceeds 99%. Donor site complications with ALT flap selections are low. A meta-analysis that evaluated donor site morbidity of ALT flaps in head and neck reconstruction demonstrated an

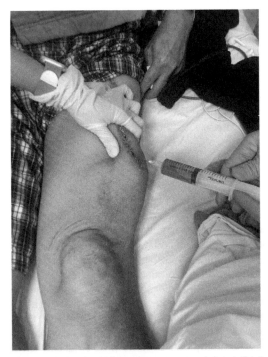

Fig. 10. Aspiration of seroma at anterolateral thigh (ALT) flap donor site.

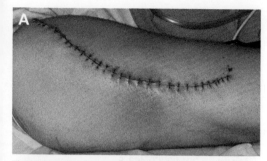

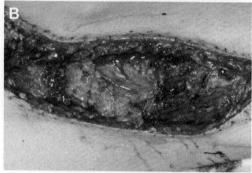

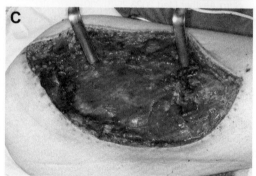

Fig. 11. Necrosis of rectus femoris muscle. (*A*) Redness and tenderness at thigh noticed at postoperative review appointment. (*B*) Ischemic muscle noticed upon surgical exploration of previous wound. (*C*) Ischemic rectus femoris excised.

overall hematoma or seroma rate of approximately 2% (**Fig. 10**), infection rate of approximately 3.6%, and wound dehiscence rate of 4.1%.[16] Therefore, complications and their subsequent management are largely related to flap indication, recipient site characteristics, and patient comorbidities.[17–22]

In our experience, 85% of the ALT donor site could be closed primarily while 15% required skin grafting. The average flap width for the former was 7.4 cm; the latter, 9.5 cm. In addition to the aforementioned general complications, 2 patients developed painful neuroma at the donor site. Pain was immediately relieved after neuroma excision. Temporary leg weakness was present in 2%, 1%, 3%, respectively, and 1% in patients with no VL muscle taken, small cuff of muscle,

half of VL muscle, and whole muscle, respectively.[23] Necrosis of RF muscle is a relatively rare but severe complication with less than a handful of cases reported so far (**Fig. 11**). In the majority (86%) of the patients, RF is supplied entirely or partially by the descending branch of LCFA, which is harvested for ALT flap.[24] When the major branch to the muscle is visualized at the proximal end of the pedicle, it should be preserved whenever possible. Upon closure, excessive tension over the RF muscle upon should be strictly avoided.

CLINICS CARE POINTS

- The ALT flap can be harvested as a chimeric flap with VL muscle.
- The motor nerve to the VL can often be spared with careful dissection away from the vascular pedicle; however, it can be harvested with the flap when indicated for nerve reconstruction at the recipient site.
- The RF branch can be used as the donor vessel for a second free flap.
- When multiple sizable perforators are identified, the ALT flap can be divided to create multiple skin islands, which can be used for reconstruction or a potential monitoring segment when the flap is buried.
- During flap harvest, caution should be exercised to avoid making the medial incision too far laterally as the perforators to the flap may be missed or inadvertently injured.
- Avoid closure of the remnant deep fascia and excessively tight closure at the donor site to avoid potential compartment syndrome and optimize wound healing.
- Pre-operative evaluation of the thigh and intra-operative evaluation of the given defect should be carefully considered as flap thickness, in particular, may impede successful reconstruction.
- When no ALT perforators are found, simple medial exploration through the same incision can lead to successful harvesting of AMT flap.
- Both ALT and AMT chimeric flaps can be harvested based on a single vascular pedicle, the descending branch of LCF system.

DISCLOSURE

The authors declare that they have no known conflict of interests or personal relationships that could have appeared to influence the work reported in this paper.

REFERENCES

1. Song YG, Chen GZ, Song YL. The free thigh flap: a new free flap concept based on the septocutaneous artery. Br J Plast Surg 1984;37(2):149–59. PMID: 6713155.

2. Koshima I, Fukuda H, Yamamoto H, et al. Free anterolateral thigh flaps for reconstruction of head and neck defects. Plast Reconstr Surg 1993;92(3):421–8. discussion 429-30. PMID: 8341740.

3. Yu P. Characteristics of the anterolateral thigh flap in a Western population and its application in head and neck reconstruction. Head Neck 2004;26(9):759–69.

4. Yu P. Reinnervated anterolateral thigh flap for tongue reconstruction. Head Neck 2004;26(12):1038–44. PMID: 15459922.

5. Kehrer A, Sachanadani NS, da Silva NPB, et al. Step-by-step guide to ultrasound-based design of alt flaps by the microsurgeon - Basic and advanced applications and device settings. J Plast Reconstr Aesthetic Surg 2020;73(6):1081–90. Epub 2019 Dec 1. PMID: 32249187.

6. Yassin AM, Kanapathy M, Khater AME, et al. Uses of Smartphone Thermal Imaging in Perforator Flaps as a Versatile Intraoperative Tool: The Microsurgeon's Third Eye. JPRAS Open 2023;38:98–108. PMID: 37753532; PMCID: PMC10518327.

7. Righini S, Festa BM, Bonanno MC, et al. Dynamic tongue reconstruction with innervated gracilis musculocutaneos flap after total glossectomy. Laryngoscope 2019;129(1):76–81. Epub 2018 Oct 16. PMID: 30325032.

8. Heredero S, Falguera-Uceda MI, Sanjuan-Sanjuan A, et al. Chimeric profunda artery perforator-gracilis flap: A computed tomographic angiography study and case report. Microsurgery 2021;41(3):250–7.

9. Jeong WH, Lee WJ, Roh TS, et al. Long-term functional outcomes after total tongue reconstruction: Consideration of flap types, volume, and functional results. Microsurgery 2017;37(3):190–6. Epub 2015 Jun 29. PMID: 26118978.

10. Yu P, Hanasono MM, Skoracki RJ, et al. Pharyngoesophageal reconstruction with the anterolateral thigh flap after total laryngopharyngectomy. Cancer 2010;116(7):1718–24.

11. Su YR, Ganry L, Ozturk C, et al. Fibula Flap Reconstruction for the Mandible: Why It Is Still the Workhorse? Atlas Oral Maxillofac Surg Clin North Am 2023;31(2):121–7.

12. Yu P, Selber J. Perforator patterns of the anteromedial thigh flap. Plast Reconstr Surg 2011;128(3):151e–7e.

13. Yu P, Selber J, Liu J. Reciprocal dominance of the anterolateral and anteromedial thigh flap perforator anatomy. Ann Plast Surg 2013;70(6):714–6.

14. Yu P. Inverse relationship of the anterolateral and anteromedial thigh flap perforator anatomy. J Reconstr Microsurg 2014;30(7):463–8.

15. Corbitt C, Skoracki RJ, Yu P, et al. Free flap failure in head and neck reconstruction. Head Neck 2014;36(10):1440–5.

16. Niu Z, Chen Y, Li Y, et al. Comparison of donor site morbidity between anterolateral thigh and radial forearm free flaps for head and neck reconstruction: a systematic review and meta-analysis. J Craniofac Surg 2021;32(5):1706–11.

17. De Ravin E, Barrette LX, Carey RM, et al. Association of head and neck anatomic zones with microvascular reconstruction outcomes. Facial Plast Surg Aesthet Med 2023;25(3):200–5.

18. Lin PC, Kuo PJ, Kuo SCH, et al. Risk factors associated with postoperative complications of free anterolateral thigh flap placement in patients with head and neck cancer: Analysis of propensity score-matched cohorts. Microsurgery 2020;40(5):538–44.

19. Hanasono MM, Zevallos JP, Skoracki RJ, et al. A prospective analysis of bony versus soft-tissue reconstruction for posterior mandibular defects. Plast Reconstr Surg 2010;125(5):1413–21.

20. Hanasono MM, Silva AK, Yu P, et al. A comprehensive algorithm for oncologic maxillary reconstruction. Plast Reconstr Surg 2013;131(1):47–60.

21. Hanasono MM, Silva A, Skoracki RJ, et al. Skull base reconstruction: an updated approach. Plast Reconstr Surg 2011;128(3):675–86.

22. Chao AH, Yu P, Skoracki RJ, et al. Microsurgical reconstruction of composite scalp and calvarial defects in patients with cancer: a 10-year experience. Head Neck 2012;34(12):1759–64.

23. Hanasono MM, Skoracki RJ, Yu P. A prospective study of donor-site morbidity after anterolateral thigh fasciocutaneous and myocutaneous free flap harvest in 220 patients. Plast Reconstr Surg 2010;125:209.

24. Zhan Y, Zhu H, Geng P, et al. Revisiting the blood supply of the rectus femoris: a case report and computed tomography angiography study. Ann Plast Surg 2020;85(4):419–23. PMID: 31913901.

The Role of Deep Inferior Epigastric Perforator and Thoracodorsal Artery Perforator Flaps in Head and Neck Reconstruction

Luís Vieira, MD, MSc[a],*, Andres Rodriguez-Lorenzo, MD, PhD[b,c]

KEYWORDS

- Deep inferior epigastric perforator flap • Thoracodorsal artery perforator flap
- Head and neck reconstruction • Perforator flap

KEY POINTS

- Deep inferior epigastric perforator flap is indicated in head and neck reconstruction for large defects where tissue bulk is required to seal death space.
- Thoracodorsal artery perforator flap is indicated in head and neck reconstruction for complex defects where both bony reconstruction and large soft tissue reconstructions are needed.
- The morbidity of both donor sites is low in terms of complications and sequela of flap harvest.

INTRODUCTION/HISTORY/DEFINITIONS/BACKGROUND

Head and neck reconstruction has known a great advance in terms of tissue replacement. The evolution of our knowledge of anatomy and angiosomes has allowed a better selection of the tissues transferred to reconstruct each defect. Perforator flaps are an evolution of microsurgery, aiming at the reduction of donor site morbidity and refinement of the transferred tissue.

Deep inferior epigastric perforator (DIEP) flap was first described by Koshima and Soeda in 1989.[1] DIEP flap allows the transfer of a large surface of skin and fat with a long pedicle with a favorable caliber with minimal donor site morbidity. This has made this flap the gold standard for autologous breast reconstruction. However, its use in head and neck is not so widespread.[2]

Thoracodorsal artery perforator (TDAP) flap was first described by Angrigiani in 1995.[3] The subscapular system, including the thoracodorsal system from which this flap derives, provides the widest array of soft tissue and osseous flaps, as well as chimeric options. Its advantages include a long pedicle, independently mobile tissue components, relative sparing from atherosclerosis, and minimal donor site morbidity.

In this article, we explore indications for the use of DIEP and TDAP flaps. A literature review and a case report are presented for each flap.

---

[a] Department of Plastic, Reconstructive and Aesthetic Surgery, Central Lisbon University Hospital, Lisboa, Portugal; [b] Department of Plastic and Maxillofacial Surgery, Uppsala University Hospital, VO. Plastik och Käkkirurgi, ing 85, 9 v, Akademiska Sjukhuset, Uppsala 75185, Sweden; [c] Department of Surgical Sciences, Uppsala University, Uppsala, Sweden
* Corresponding author.
E-mail addresses: Luisgsvieira.lv@gmail.com; 72655@ulssjose.min-saude.pt

Oral Maxillofacial Surg Clin N Am 36 (2024) 463–474
https://doi.org/10.1016/j.coms.2024.07.012
1042-3699/24/© 2024 Elsevier Inc. All rights are reserved, including those for text and data mining, AI training, and similar technologies.

DISCUSSION
Deep Inferior Epigastric Perforator Flap in Head and Neck Reconstruction

Preoperative planning and anatomy
The DIEP flap is harvested from the abdomen, based on perforators from the deep inferior epigastric vessels. The design of the skin paddle can be tailor made to the defect, although a horizontal scar is usually preferred as it is more easily concealed (**Fig. 1**). The periumbilical perforators are usually of larger caliber. Preoperative angio-computed tomography is usually used to map the best perforators in terms of caliber, location, and intramuscular course. After perforator selection, the pedicle is dissected in its intramuscular course through the rectus abdominis muscle, sparing this muscle and its motor nerves for prevention of donor site morbidity (**Fig. 2**). The pedicle can be dissected to its origin from the external iliac vessels providing up to 12 cm of length.

Indications and contraindications
DIEP flaps are indicated when a large volume of tissue is needed, or when a large skin paddle is intended for resurfacing.

A recent systematic review[2] described the main indications in the literature - glossectomy defects, orbitomaxillary defects, scalp and calvaria defects, and anterior and lateral skull base defects.

Glossectomy defects Many authors have described the merits of DIEP flaps for oral reconstruction. In 2000, Koshima described a multi-lobe "accordion" thin flap based on periumbilical perforators allowing tongue and floor of the mouth reconstruction with good functional outcomes, besides reduction of

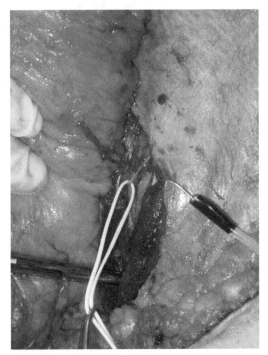

Fig. 2. After perforator selection in the suprafascial plane, the muscular fascia is opened and the perforator is dissected in its intramuscular course. Care is taken to preserve the nerve branches, as seen in the yellow loop.

salivary fistulas by dead space obliteration by the large volume of the flap in the neck.[4] In 2013, Yano[5] reported a pediatric tongue reconstruction with a DIEP flap, making use of its pliability and its volume for death space obliteration, with a good result in diet and speech function. The same author[6] approached the issue of death space obliteration in intraoral resections with neck communication with the use of DIEP flaps with 2 skin paddles, one of them deeptihelialized for that purpose. These authors avoided other muscle flaps for this indication as in these cases, the patients had a special interest in avoiding muscle weakening in the abdominal wall because of professional purposes. Zhang[7] presented 12 cases of head and neck reconstruction with DIEP flaps, 6 of which were glossectomy defects, of which 5 resumed oral feeding and decannulation in an average of 16 days. This series uses this flap in head and neck reconstruction in males only, as this flap is too bulky in females, and the vessels are also smaller, when compared to other options as the anterolateral thigh (ALT) flap. In 2006, Woodworht and colleagues[8] presented their experience with abdominal muscle sparing free flaps for head and neck reconstruction, of which 11 were DIEP flaps for partial or total glossectomy reconstruction, total

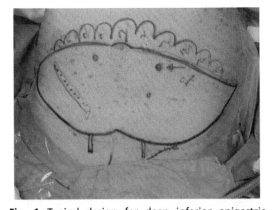

Fig. 1. Typical design for deep inferior epigastric perforator (DIEP) harvesting. The horizontal skin paddle allows concealing of the scar in the lower abdomen as in abdominoplasty. Preoperative Angio-computed tomography (CT) allows location of the more suitable perforators for the reconstruction needs.

parotidectomy and pinna reconstruction, and cranio-facial reconstruction. The authors describe no sequela in the donor site.

In 2012, Burgueño presented a case series of 7 total glossectomies reconstructed with DIEP flaps.[9] The feeding outcome was poor, in which 57,1% of the patients required a permanent gastrostomy. On the other hand, speech was considered intelligible in 85% of the cases. For total glossectomy reconstruction, this group used vertically oriented fusiform DIEP flaps on zone I. No major surgical complications were observed, and there were no sequelae in donor site.

Beausang[10] described their experience with DIEP flaps in 9 cases of glossectomy defects reconstruction. For this defect, they also used a vertically oriented skin paddle based in zone I. The authors underlie the low morbidity profile of this donor site.

In the largest series to date, Masià[11] presented the reconstruction of 100 patients with DIEP flaps for head and neck reconstruction. The authors use a variation of the flap, the extended DIEP flap, in which the skin paddle is obliquely oriented from a periumbilical perforator in an axis to the scapula tip. This design allows avoidance of hair bearing skin, and the use of a thinner skin paddle, when compared to the classical horizontal DIEP. This flap also has the advantage of a longer pedicle, when compared to the ALT, for example, the location of the defects is not presented in this study.

Orbitomaxillary defects When dealing with orbitomaxillary defects, DIEP flaps can be indicated because of the adequate bulk and versatility for large 3-dimensional reconstructions. In 2000, Marchetti[12] described their transition from musculocutaneous to perforator flaps in skull base and orbitomaxillary reconstruction. They used 1 DIEP flap for skull base reconstruction and used its versatility for sealing dead space and reconstruction of different surfaces with de-epithelialized segments and paddles of skin. They reinforce the maintenance of the volume of the reconstruction because no muscle atrophy occurred afterward.

In 2006, Sekido[13] used a DIEP flap with 2 segments of costal cartilage for midface reconstruction. The costal cartilages were used to reconstruct the orbital floor and the zygomaticomaxillary buttress, while the skin paddle of the flap was used to resurface the nasal lining and the palate. In this case, patient's body habitus precluded the use of Rectus Abdominis Myocutaneous (RAMC) because of excessive bulk. The postoperative course was uneventful. The simultaneous vascularization of the costal cartilages by the connection of the DIEP pedicle to the 8th intercostal pedicle is used for such reconstruction.

Guerra[14] described their experience with 12 DIEP flaps for head and neck reconstruction, of which 3 were for maxilla reconstruction. These authors underlie how reconstruction with fasciocutaneous flaps can be superior to musculocutaneous flaps in terms of imaging surveillance, as the fat enhances brightly on MRI T1-weighted images, allowing identification of early recurrences.

In 2014, Zhang[15] presented their experience with 8 DIEP flaps for skull base reconstruction, for which they found similar rates of reconstruction complications as compared to musculocutaneous free flaps. They recommend DIEP flap for large 3-dimensional reconstructions.

Miyamoto[16] described their evolution from RAMC to DIEP flap for maxilla reconstruction. They point the unpredictable muscle atrophy, shortage of pedicle length, and donor-site morbidity as their main reasons for the change. In this 10-patient cohort, the authors use a vertically oriented *peanut shaped* design, further divided in different skin paddles for orbital floor reconstruction, nasal lining, and palate reconstruction. De-epithelialized segments are used for dead space obliteration. The maintenance of the volume of the flap in the long-term makes its inset more predictable and avoids reoperations for flap repositioning.

Clemens[17] described buried DIEP flaps in a delayed setting for contour reconstruction in 6 patients. Their experience was successful in different head and neck locations. The DIEP flap in this setting could later be revised and transferred on pedicles for better volume restoration, even in the setting of radiotherapy, proving more valuable than alloplastic reconstruction.

Scalp and calvaria defects In 1999, Ağaoğlu[18] reported their experience of hair micrografting of a freely transferred pre-expanded DIEP flap for treatment of cicatricial alopecia. Although the DIEP flaps successfully replaced the scarred scalp, the experience with hair micrografting was not successful due to infection and fat necrosis.

For posterior neck reconstruction, Margulis[19] presented a case of excision and reconstruction of a giant melanocytic nevus with a pre-expanded DIEP flap. In this case, after the transfer, the flap was re-expanded in the recipient site. The lesion was almost totally excised, and the aesthetic result was good.

Guerra[14] also reported 4 cases of reconstruction of large defects of calvaria post oncological resection, with good outcomes overall.

In their work in 2010, Chang[20] describe their algorithm for scalp and calvaria reconstruction, in which they prefer myocutaneous free flaps for cases of infection and need for dead space obliteration. In this 12 cases series, they used 1 DIEP flap for a scalp reconstruction.

Kostakoğlu[21] presented their experience with DIEP flaps in 2 scalp reconstructions. They used an extended DIEP flap, with an oblique orientation, as described by Taylor. The largest defect was 30x18 cm.

In the setting of a cranioplasty infection with a resulting large bony and soft tissue defect, Slater[22] described the use of a bipedicled DIEP flap. Bilateral anastomosis to the superficial temporal vessels provided a rich blood supply, which allowed a 2-stage soft tissue and bony reconstruction.

Table 1 summarizes the results described in the literature from the use of DIEP flap in head and neck reconstruction. The morbidity from the donor site is low, namely in terms of abdominal wall weakness. The rates of partial and total necrosis of the transferred flap are also low, which shows the feasibility of this flap for head and neck reconstruction (**Box 1**).

CASE STUDY/PRESENTATION

A 47-year-old woman sustained a necrotizing fasciitis in the neck. In the acute setting, after serial debridement, the defect was initially reconstructed with split thickness skin graft. Due to neck retraction and unstable scar, it was decided to replace the skin graft with a DIEP flap connected to the right-side transverse cervical artery and external jugular vein. After 2 secondary corrections including flap debulking the patient achieved a satisfactory result (**Fig. 3**).

THORACODORSAL ARTERY PERFORATOR FLAP IN HEAD AND NECK RECONSTRUCTION
Preoperative Planning and Anatomy

There is not routinely need for imaging of the donor site. Preoperative evaluation of the thoracodorsal nerve function indicates integrity of the thoracodorsal pedicle in case of previous surgeries in the axilla. This flap can be raised either in lateral decubitus or dorsal decubitus with proper shoulder flexion. Thoracodorsal perforators can usually be found 8 cm distal do the armpit and 2 cm behind the latissimus dorsi anterior border in a subfascial plane on the latissimus dorsi muscle. A preoperative doppler signal can map such perforator. Regular distal to proximal perforator dissection is then performed in its intramuscular course. For inclusion of the scapula tip, the space between the latissimus dorsi and the teres major muscles is explored. The scapula tip and its nourishing angular vessels can be found in such space

(**Fig. 4**). After evaluation of the reconstruction needs, both bone muscle and skin paddles can be harvested in 1 vascular pedicle. A template of the defect is useful for proper flap design (**Fig. 5**).

Indications and Contraindications

The TDAP flap has been described in the literature for use as a purely fasciocutaneous flap, or as chimeric flap with other components, namely bone from scapula.

Complex oromandibular reconstructions with oral, extraoral skin, and bony defects have been successfully reconstructed with chimeric scapular and TDAP flaps.[23] Such flap avoids the need for 2 free flaps, allows bony reconstruction, and is superior to the fibula flap in terms of soft tissue reconstruction.

Pau described the thoracodorsal, perforator-scapular flap based on the angular artery in 2019.[24] In this study, 5 patients with extensive oromandibular tumors were treated. The TDAP skin paddle was used for intraoral reconstruction, and the scapula tip osteotomized and used for mandible reconstruction. The authors underlie the virtue of the subscapular system to avoid multiple free flaps for extensive defects. Besides, the avoidance of a musculocutaneous flap through the harvest of a purely perforator-based skin paddle allows a less bulky reconstruction.

In a study focused on donor site morbidity and quality of life,[25] 20 cases of maxillomandibular reconstruction are described using a chimeric TDAP and scapula tip flap for post-oncologic reconstruction or osteoradionecrosis reconstruction. Eighteen cases were mandibular reconstructions, and 2 cases maxillary reconstruction. The average size of the harvested skin paddle was 86 cm^2 ($\pm$49.8; range 16–200 cm^2), and the length of the harvested bone graft ranged from 4 to 12 cm and the width from 2.4 to 3 cm. Since the skin is harvested without the underlying muscle when using the TDAP-scap-aa (Thoracodorsal, Perforator-Scapular Flap Based on the Angular Artery) technique, a comfortable structure lining owing to the reduced soft tissue thickness and volume is possible. This is particularly important if the tongue, the pharynx, and/or the palate are part of the soft tissue reconstruction. The data of the study conclude that the donor-site morbidity after scapular free flap harvesting is low 1 year after flap harvesting. The overall quality of life was found to be in the upper third compared to the norm population.

In another study, the donor site morbidity of the TDAP was compared to that of radial forearm in cases of oral and oropharyngeal reconstruction[26]

Table 1
Complications related to deep inferior epigastric perforator flap in head and neck reconstruction

Author	n	Donor Site Infection	Dehiscence	Outcome	Abdominal Wall Weakness/Bulging/Hernia	Recipient Site Partial Necrosis	Total Necrosis	Dehiscence	Infection	Fistula	Reintervention (Emergent/Revision)	CSF Leakage	Outcome	Follow up (Months)
Koshima et al,[4] 2000	1	0	0	NA	0	0	0	0	0	0	0	0	0	NA
Yano et al,[4] 2013	1	0	0	Full part in gymnastics	0	0	0	0	0	0	0	0	Understandable speech, regular diet	12
Yano et al,[6] 2009	2	0	0	0	1 transient weakening	0	0	1	1	0	1	0	Regular diet and speech	18
Zhang et al,[7] 2009	12	0	0	NA	NA	0	1	1	0	1	0	0	5/6 resumed total oral feeding. 5/6 intelligible speech	NA
Woodworth et al,[8] 2006	11	0	1	NA	0	0	0	0	0	0	0	0	NA	21
López-Arcas et al,[9] 2012	7	0	0	NA	0	0	1	1	0	0	0	0	Permanent gastrostomy - 57.1%. Intelligible speech-85.7%	NA
Beausang et al,[10] 2003	13	0	0	NA	0	0	1	0	0	0	0	0	5 patients total glossectomies - intelligible speech	NA
Masià et al,[11] 2011	102	0	0	NA	0	3	0	0	0	0	0	0	NA	NA
Marchetti et al,[12] 2002	1	0	0	NA	0	0	0	0	0	0	0	1	NA	6

(continued on next page)

Table 1
(continued)

Author	n	Donor Site			Recipient Site									
		Infection	Dehiscence	Outcome	Abdominal Wall Weakness/ Bulging/ Hernia	Partial Necrosis	Total Necrosis	Dehiscence	Infection	Fistula	Reintervention (Emergent/ Revision)	CSF Leakage	Outcome	Follow up (Months)
Sekido et al,[13] 2006	1	0	0	NA	0	0	0	0	0	0	0	0	Good contour. Regular diet	6
Guerra et al,[14] 2005	12	2	0	NA	0	1	1	0	0	0	4 for debulking	0	NA	NA
Zhang et al,[15] 2014	8	0	0	NA	0	0	0	0	2	0	0	2	NA	10
Miyamoto et al,[16] 2019	10	0	0	NA	0	0	0	0	4	0	1 for arterial thrombosis. 2 revisionary surgeries	0	NA	13
Clemens et al,[17] 2009	6	0	0	NA	0	0	0	0	0	0	3 recontouring	0	Patient-reported good to excellent	16
Ağaoğlu et al,[18] 1999	1	0	0	NA	0	0	0	0	1	0	0	0	NA	NA
Margulis et al,[19] 2010	1	0	0	NA	0	0	0	0	0	0	1 re-expansion	0	Excellent aesthetic result	NA
Chang et al,[20] 2010	1	0	0	NA	0	0	0	0	0	0	0	0	NA	NA
Kostakoğlu et al,[21] 1998	2	0	0	NA	0	0	0	0	0	0	0	0	NA	36
Slater et al,[23] 2014	1	0	0	NA	0	0	0	0	0	0	0	0	NA	NA
Total (n/%)	193	2 (1%)	1 (0.5%)	NA	1 transient	1 (0.5%)	6 (3%)	3 (1.5%)	8 (4%)	1 (0.5%)	2 emergent/7 revision	3 (1.5%)	NA	NA

Abbreviation: NA, not available.

Advantages	Disadvantages
Long pedicle	Tedious intramuscular dissection
Two team approach	Color mismatch
Reliable large skin paddle	
Bulk for death space obliteration	
Low donor site morbidity	
Potential for flap thinning	

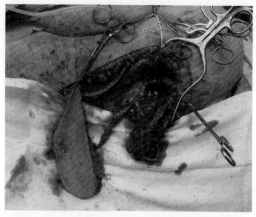

Fig. 4. Intraoperative picture of the thoracodorsal artery perforator (TDAP) and scapula tip flap. Note the perforator nourishing the skin paddle, and the vascular pedicle to the scapula tip bone, which join and continue as the thoracodorsal vessels.

and had a favorable result in terms of scar quality and impact in quality of life.

For extensive parotidectomy defects with facial nerve resection with or without skin defect, Bedarida and colleagues, 2020 present 8 cases of chimeric reconstruction with TDAP flap and vascularized thoracodorsal nerve to bridge the facial nerve defect. The thoracodorsal perforator was used to vascularize either a skin paddle (5 cases) or a fatty tissue island (3 cases), depending on the requirements of each case. In this case series, 6 patients achieved a House Brackman score of IV, and 2 had a score of III. The best results were achieved for eye reinnervation, with all patients achieving total eye closure.[27]

A new application of the chimeric scapula tip TDAP is described[28] for subtotal and total tongue reconstruction. In this 3 cases series, the skin paddle is used for tongue reconstruction, and a segment of 3 to 4 5 cm of scapula tip is used to reconstruct the floor of the mouth. Although all patients kept dependence on gastrostomy for feeding, the speech results were promising. The authors suggest that the soft tissue component of the flap shows adequate thickness, width, and pliability to create the neotongue and separate the neck from oral cavity. At the same time, the scapular tip exhibits ideal morphology to suit the floor of the mouth space while maintaining flap position over time.

A variation in skin paddle orientation has also been explored for TDAP harvesting. In this study,

the flaps are designed in a horizontal orientation, aiming to decrease donor site morbidity in terms of scar widening, and aiming to include perforator from the transverse branch of the thoracodorsal pedicle. Twelve cases of head and neck reconstruction were included in this series. Of the 40 perforators dissected in this series, 6 derived from the transverse branch.

To reduce cutaneous scarring in the axilla for cosmetic reasons, Tawa[29] described a horizontal skin paddle for TDAP harvesting, with good outcome in a hemi glossectomy reconstruction in a young female.

The specific subset of septocutaneous TDAP (TDAP-sc) flaps is explored by Miyamoto.[30] In this article, 6 head and neck defects are reconstructed with purely septocutaneous perforator TDAP flaps. When one large septocutaneous perforator was found with color Doppler ultrasonography, elevation of the TDAP-sc flap was attempted. The scapula was simultaneously harvested based on the angular branch in 3 patients who underwent immediate mandibular reconstruction. Based on this study and on this group's

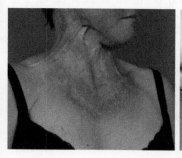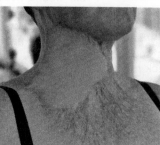

Fig. 3. Left, preoperative photo of the patient after split thickness skin graft. On the right, 8 years follow-up photo after DIEP flap reconstruction.

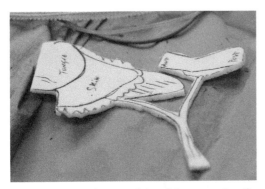

Fig. 5. Intraoperative template of the reconstruction needs to be harvested in the flap.

experience, the prevalence of sizable septocutaneous perforator from the thoracodorsal pedicle is 50%. The main advantages of such flaps are the easier perforator dissection without intramuscular course, diminished risk of lesion to the thoracodorsal nerve, and the chance to have a venous supercharge through the inclusion of the lateral thoracic vein in the flap. In this study, 6 large TDAP-sc flaps ($\geq$20 cm long) completely survived.

For the treatment of sequela after limited maxillectomy/anteromedial maxillectomy plus radiotherapy and intraarterial chemotherapy, Sarukawa[31] present chimeric TDAP flap and scapula tip. For that purpose, the authors designed a 3-part flap spindle-shaped skin paddles, 2 to rebuild lateral nasal cavity wall and oral vestibule and the third providing a dermal fat pad for cheek augmentation. The scapula tip was used for zygomatic reconstruction. In this difficult cohort, all patients needed surgical revisions, mostly for some defects of the orbital floor or zygomatic prominence.

The versatility of the subscapular system is explored for secondary reconstruction of complex middle and lower face traumatic defects.[32] In this case series, 3 patients were reconstructed with chimeric flaps that included scapular bone based on the angular artery and TDAP fasciocutaneous tissue island components. Two other cases are presented in which a musculocutaneous latissimus dorsi flap is used. The indications were: contour deformity at the supraorbital rim, persistent maxillary defect, large oronasal fistula, and soft tissue deficiency at the nose and upper lip.

Lee[33] presents 5 cases of extensive capillary malformations (CM) in the head and neck region successfully treated with radical excision and reconstruction with fasciocutaneous TDAP flaps. The average size of harvested flaps was 146.8 cm. All flaps survived without recurrence of CM on the skin paddle of the transferred flap.

The patients achieved high levels of aesthetic restoration and satisfaction.

Bach[34] describes oropharyngeal and soft palate reconstruction in 9 patients with TDAP flap, as an alternative to radial forearm or ALT flaps. Besides the low donor site morbidity, they report good functional results—the speech was evaluated as "clearly understood" in 7 patients, and feeding was resumed at a mean of 15 days.

In a non-head and neck specific study comparing single versus multiple perforator TDAP flap, Karaaltin[35] found a higher prevalence of flap related complication in the single perforator group, namely venous drainage issues. From the 87 patients studied, 16 were head and neck reconstructions.

In 2 cases of contour deformity in the temporal and masseteric region caused by trigeminal nerve denervation, Mun[36] described proper correction with the transfer of dual paddle thoracodorsal perforator adipofascial free flaps.

Table 2 summarizes the results described in the literature from the use of thoracodorsal perforator flap in head and neck reconstruction. The morbidity from the donor site is low, namely in terms of upper limb function. The reconstruction outcomes are also good (**Box 2**).

CASE STUDY/PRESENTATION

A 69-year-old female patient with previous medical history of colon and uterus cancer, hypothyroidism, moderate smoking habits, and limited mobility, presented with an advanced squamous cell carcinoma in the floor of the mouth with infiltration of the left tongue and destruction of left mandible, classified as T4aN0M0. After discussion at the institution's Head and Neck Tumor Board, the patient underwent mandibulectomy, hemiglossectomy, and neck dissection (**Fig. 6**). Mandible and tongue reconstruction were performed with a chimeric scapula tip and TDAP free flap (**Fig. 7**).

During the postoperative period, the patient developed an infection in the recipient site that responded well to antibiotic treatment. The patient was discharged home after 5 weeks (**Fig. 8**). Stable wound healing occurred in both donor and recipient sites. Postoperative analysis of the tumor resection showed radical resection of the tumor with close margin, upgrading the tumor stage to pT3N3bM0. Postoperative radiotherapy (66 Gy) was administered, and the patient received a gastrostomy for nutrition.

At 7 months postoperative, the patient developed a metastasis in the right neck, underwent modified neck dissection, and passed away 14 months postoperatively.

Table 2
Complications related to thoracodorsal perforator flap in head and neck reconstruction

Author	n	Donor Site					Recipient Site						
		Hematoma	Infection	Dehiscence	Skin Grafting	Outcome	Partial Necrosis	Total Necrosis	Dehiscence	Infection	Fistula	Reintervention	Outcome
Wallner et al,[25] 2022	20	0	0	0	0	Mean DASH - 21.74	0	0	0	0	0	0	NA
Bedarida et al,[27] 2020	8	0	0	0	0	NA	0	0	0	0	0	0	6 patients – HB IV; 2 patients – HB III
Ferrari et al,[28] 2020	3	0	0	0	0	NA	0	0	0	0	0	0	NA
Tawa et al,[29] 2019	1	0	0	0	0	NA	0	0	0	0	0	0	NA
Miyamoto et al,[30] 2019	6	0	0	0	0	NA	0	0	0	2	1	0	NA
Sarukawa et al,[31] 2017	2	0	0	0	0	NA	1	0	0	1	0	0	NA
Shaw et al,[23] 2015	2	0	0	0	0	NA	0	0	0	0	0	0	NA
Bach et al,[26] 2015	7	0	0	0	0	Global satisfaction 9.3; PSAS 9; Vancouver 2.7; OSAS 14.1	0	0	0	0	0	0	NA
Stalder et al,[32] 2015	3	0	0	0	0	NA	0	0	0	0	0	1	NA
Lee et al,[33] 2016	5	0	0	0	1	NA	1	0	1	0	0	1	NA
Bach et al,[34] 2015	9	0	0	0	0	NA	0	0	1	1	1	2	NA
Chepeha et al,[37] 2010	20	0	0	0	0	NA	0	0	0	0	0	0	NA
Mun et al,[36] 2006	2	0	0	0	0	NA	0	0	0	0	0	0	NA
Total (n/%)	88	0	0	0	1 (1.1%)	NA	2 (2.2%)	0	2 (2.2%)	4 (4.5%)	2 (2.2%)	4 (4.5%)	NA

Abbreviations: HB, house brackman, NA, not available, OSAS, observer scar assessment scale; PSAS, patient scar assessment scale.

Box 2
Advantages and disadvantages

Advantages	Disadvantages
Chimeric flap (Fasciocutaneous, scapula bone segment, muscle – latissimus dorsi, serratus, thoracodorsal nerve)	Eventual need for decubitus change, depending on surgeon experience
Mobility between elements of the chimeric flaps	Color mismatch
Long pedicle	Tedious intramuscular dissection of musculocutaneous perforators
Subscapular pedicle spared from arteriosclerosis	Limited bone stock
Low donor site morbidity	
Constant anatomy	

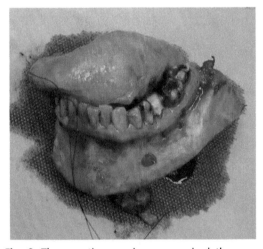

Fig. 6. The resection specimen comprised the mandible from angle to angle, subtotal glossectomy, and floor of the mouth.

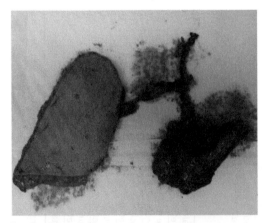

Fig. 7. Chimeric flap on the subscapular system comprising scapula tip and thoracodorsal perforator flap.

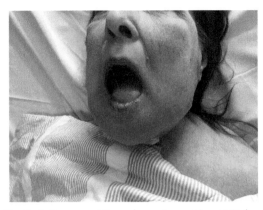

Fig. 8. Follow-up at 5 weeks postoperative period.

SUMMARY
Indications

DIEP Flap in Head and Neck	TDAP Flap in Head and Neck
Large surface defect	Complex defects requiring both bony and large soft tissue reconstruction
Large volume defect requiring death space sealing	Comorbid patient with peripheral artery disease
Patient preference for donor site with hidden scar	Other donor sites exhausted (example ALT)

CLINICS CARE POINTS

- DIEP flap is a reliable flap with low donor site morbidity.
- DIEP flaps have a large well-vascularized skin paddle for large surface defect reconstruction.
- DIEP flaps allow the tailoring of the flap's bulkiness by different designs and potential thinning.
- TDAP is a soft and pliable fasciocutaneous flap with the hypothesis to add chimeric components (bone, muscle, and nerve) for complex reconstruction.
- Donor site morbidity is low – hidden scar, no muscle loss of function, usually no healing problems, large flaps can be harvested, and the donor site closed primarily.
- The subscapular system is less affected from arteriosclerosis in comorbid patients, namely with severe peripheral vascular disease.

- As a purely fasciocutaneous flap, useful when other donor sites (eg, ALT) are exhausted.
- Perforator flap dissection requires proper surgical technique for small vessel dissection in intramuscular course.

DISCLOSURE

The authors have no financial interest to declare in relation to the content of this article. No funding was received for this study.

REFERENCES

1. Koshima I, Soeda S. Inferior epigastric artery skin flaps without rectus abdominis muscle. Br J Plast Surg 1989;42(6):645–8.
2. Mayo-Yáñez M, Rodríguez-Pérez E, Chiesa-Estomba CM, et al. Deep inferior epigastric artery perforator free flap in head and neck reconstruction: a systematic review. J Plast Reconstr Aesthetic Surg 2021;74(4):718–29.
3. Angrigiani C, Grilli D, Siebert J. Latissimus dorsi musculocutaneous flap without muscle. Plast Reconstr Surg 1995;96(7):1608–14.
4. Koshima I, Hosoda M, Moriguchi T, et al. New multi-lobe "accordion" flaps for three-dimensional reconstruction of wide, full-thickness defects in the oral floor. Ann Plast Surg 2000;45(2):187–92.
5. Yano T, Okazaki M, Kawaguchi R, et al. Tongue reconstruction with minimal donor site morbidity using a deep inferior epigastric perforator (DIEP) free flap in a 6-year-old girl. Microsurgery 2013;33(6):487–90.
6. Yano T, Sakuraba M, Asano T, et al. Head and neck reconstruction with the deep inferior epigastric perforator flap: a report of two cases. Microsurgery 2009;29(4):287–92.
7. Zhang B, Li D-Z, Xu Z-G, et al. Deep inferior epigastric artery perforator free flaps in head and neck reconstruction. Oral Oncol 2009;45(2):116–20.
8. Woodworth BA, Gillespie MB, Day T, et al. Muscle-sparing abdominal free flaps in head and neck reconstruction. Head Neck 2006;28(9):802–7.
9. López-Arcas JM, Arias J, Morán MJ, et al. The deep inferior epigastric artery perforator (DIEAP) flap for total glossectomy reconstruction. J Oral Maxillofac Surg 2012;70(3):740–7.
10. Beausang ES, McKay D, Brown DH, et al. Deep inferior epigastric artery perforator flaps in head and neck reconstruction. Ann Plast Surg 2003;51(6):561–3.
11. Masià J, Sommario M, Cervelli D, et al. Extended deep inferior epigastric artery perforator flap for head and neck reconstruction: a clinical experience with 100 patients. Head Neck 2011;33(9):1328–34.
12. Marchetti C, Gessaroli M, Cipriani R, et al. Use of "perforator flaps" in skull base reconstruction after tumor resection. Plast Reconstr Surg 2002;110(5):1303–9.
13. Sekido M, Yamamoto Y, Makino S. Maxillary reconstruction using a free Deep Inferior Epigastric Perforator (DIEP) flap combined with vascularised costal cartilages. J Plast Reconstr Aesthetic Surg 2006;59(12):1350–4.
14. Guerra AB, Lyons GD, Dupin CL, Metzinger SE. Advantages of perforator flaps in reconstruction of complex defects of the head and neck. Ear Nose Throat J 2005;84(7):441–7.
15. Zhang B, Wan JH, Wan HF, et al. Free perforator flap transfer for reconstruction of skull base defects after resection of advanced recurrent tumor. Microsurgery 2014;34(8):623–8.
16. Miyamoto S, Arikawa M, Fujiki M. Deep inferior epigastric artery perforator flap for maxillary reconstruction. Laryngoscope 2019;129(6):1325–9.
17. Clemens MW, Davison SP. Buried deep inferior epigastric perforator flaps for complex head and neck contour defects. J Reconstr Microsurg 2009;25(2):81–8.
18. Ağaoğlu G, Mavili E, Kostakoglu N. Hair transplantation using a freely transferred nonhair-bearing skin flap. Ann Plast Surg 1999;43(6):649–52.
19. Margulis A, Adler N, Eyal G. Expanded deep inferior epigastric artery perforator flap for reconstruction of the posterior neck and the upper back in a child with giant congenital melanocytic nevus. J Plast Reconstr Aesthetic Surg 2010;63(9):e703–5.
20. Chang K, Lai C, Chang C, et al. Free flap options for reconstruction of complicated scalp and calvarial defects: report of a series of cases and literature review. Microsurgery 2010;30(1):13–8.
21. Kostakoğlu N, Keçik A. Deep inferior epigastric artery (DIEA) skin flap: clinical experience of 15 cases. Br J Plast Surg 1998;51(1):25–31.
22. Slater JC, Sosin M, Rodriguez ED, et al. Bilateral, bipedicled DIEP flap for staged reconstruction of cranial deformity. Craniomaxillofacial Trauma Reconstr 2014;7(4):313–7.
23. Shaw RJ, Ho MW, Brown JS. Thoracodorsal artery perforator - Scapular flap in oromandibular reconstruction with associated large facial skin defects. Br J Oral Maxillofac Surg 2015;53(6):569–71.
24. Pau M, Wallner J, Feichtinger M, et al. Free thoracodorsal, perforator-scapular flap based on the angular artery (TDAP-Scap-aa): clinical experiences and description of a novel technique for single flap reconstruction of extensive oromandibular defects. J Cranio-Maxillofacial Surg 2019;47(10):1617–25.
25. Wallner J, Rieder M, Schwaiger M, et al. Donor site morbidity and quality of life after microvascular head and neck reconstruction with a chimeric,

thoracodorsal, perforator-scapular flap based on the angular artery (TDAP-Scap-aa Flap). J Clin Med 2022;11(16). https://doi.org/10.3390/jcm11164876.

26. Bach CA, Dreyfus JF, Wagner I, et al. Comparison of radial forearm flap and thoracodorsal artery perforator flap donor site morbidity for reconstruction of oral and oropharyngeal defects in head and neck cancer. Eur Ann Otorhinolaryngol Head Neck Dis 2015;132(4):185–9.

27. Bedarida V, Qassemyar Q, Temam S, et al. Facial functional outcomes analysis after reconstruction by vascularized thoracodorsal nerve free flap following radical parotidectomy with facial nerve sacrifice. Head Neck 2020;42(5):994–1003.

28. Ferrari M, Sahovaler A, Chan HHL, et al. Scapular tip-thoracodorsal artery perforator free flap for to-tal/subtotal glossectomy defects: case series and conformance study. Oral Oncol 2020;105. https://doi.org/10.1016/j.oraloncology.2020.104660.

29. Tawa P, Foirest C, Tankéré F, et al. Tongue recon-struction by thoracodorsal perforator flap: a new har-vesting technique to reduce morbidity. Ann Chir Plast Esthet 2019;64(4):368–73.

30. Miyamoto S, Arikawa M, Kagaya Y, et al. Septocuta-neous thoracodorsal artery perforator flaps: a retro-spective cohort study. J Plast Reconstr Aesthetic Surg 2019;72(1):78–84.

31. Sarukawa S, Kamochi H, Noguchi T, et al. Free-flap surgical correction of facial deformity after antero-medial maxillectomy. J Cranio-Maxillofacial Surg 2017;45(9):1573–7.

32. Stalder M, Wise M, Dupin CL, et al. Versatility of sub-scapular chimeric free flaps in the secondary recon-struction of composite posttraumatic defects of the upper face. Craniomaxillofacial Trauma Reconstr 2015;8(1):42–9.

33. Lee DH, Pyon JK, Mun GH, et al. Reconstruction of head and neck capillary malformations with free perforator flaps for aesthetic purposes. Ann Plast Surg 2016;77(1):13–6.

34. Bach CA, Wagner I, Pigot JL, et al. Velopharyngeal function after free thoracodorsal artery perforator flap in lateral and superior oropharyngeal cancer. Eur Arch Oto-Rhino-Laryngol 2015;272(10):3019–26.

35. Karaaltin MV, Erdem A, Kuvat S, et al. Comparison of clinical outcomes between single-and multiple-perforator- based free thoracodorsal artery perfo-rator flaps: clinical experience in 87 patients. Plast Reconstr Surg 2011;128(3). https://doi.org/10.1097/PRS.0b013e318221ddd0.

36. Mun GH, Lim SY, Hyun WS, et al. Correction of tem-poro-masseteric contour deformity using the dual paddle thoracodorsal artery perforator adiposal flap. J Reconstr Microsurg 2006;22(5):335–41.

37. Chepeha DB, Khariwala SS, Chanowski EJ, et al. Thoracodorsal artery scapular tip autogenous trans-plant: vascularized bone with a long pedicle and flexible soft tissue. Arch Otolaryngol Head Neck Surg 2010;136(10):958–64.

Profunda Artery Perforator Flaps in Head and Neck Reconstruction
Anatomy, Surgical Techniques, and Evolving Applications

Rami Elmorsi, MD[a], Z-Hye Lee, MD[a], Tarek Ismail, MD[b], Rene D. Largo, MD[a],*

KEYWORDS

• Plastic surgery • Microsurgery • Dimensions • Size • Depth • Outcomes

KEY POINTS

• Profunda artery perforator (PAP) flaps offer significant volume, pliable tissue, and a discreet donor-site scar, making them particularly suitable for head and neck reconstructions, especially in patients with a lower body mass.
• The PAP flap is highly effective for reconstructive procedures such as subtotal or total glossectomy, maxillary sinus obliteration, and external cheek coverage.
• PAP flaps have certain limitations, including a small pedicle diameter, and are less suitable as chimeric flaps since the inclusion of the adductor magnus muscle component significantly reduces the pedicle length.

INTRODUCTION

Reconstructive surgeons have a plethora of options when it comes to choosing donor sites for soft-tissue flaps in head and neck reconstruction, each with its advantages and disadvantages. Certain flaps, including the radial forearm flap and the anterolateral thigh (ALT) flap, have been traditionally treated as "workhorses" due to their reliability, versatility, and suitability for various reconstructive purposes. Numerous alternatives to conventional flaps have been described for head and neck reconstruction, which not only fulfill the esthetic and functional requirements but also minimize donor-site morbidity. Examples include the ulnar artery perforator flap, the superficial circumflex iliac artery perforator flap, the lateral arm flap and its modifications, the medial sural artery perforator flap, and the profunda artery perforator (PAP) flap.[1–5] A significant advantage of the PAP flap lies in its capacity to incorporate a substantial volume of hairless, pliable skin, and fat tissue from a discrete donor site even in patients with low body mass indices, as it is frequently observed in the demography of patient with head and neck cancer.[6]

This review article endeavors to offer a comprehensive overview of the anatomic characteristics, clinical application, and pertinent recommendations for employing the PAP flap in the context of head and neck reconstruction.

HISTORIC PERSPECTIVE

Skin flaps from the posteromedial thigh emerged in 1947 when Conway and colleagues[7,8] first reported them for regional reconstruction. Later on, Song and colleagues[9] introduced the free flap variant in

a Department of Plastic Surgery, The University of Texas MD Anderson Cancer Center, 19th Floor, Pickens Tower, 1400 Pressler Street, Houston, TX 77030, USA; b Division of Plastic, Reconstructive, Aesthetic and Hand Surgery, Department of Surgery, University Hospital of Basel, Spitalstrasse 21, Basel 4031, Switzerland
* Corresponding author.
E-mail address: rdlargo@mdanderson.org

Oral Maxillofacial Surg Clin N Am 36 (2024) 475–487
https://doi.org/10.1016/j.coms.2024.07.014
1042-3699/24/Published by Elsevier Inc.

1984. However, it was not until 2001 when Angriani and colleagues[10] popularized the "adductor flap," based on the adductor magnus perforators, that the posteromedial thigh started gaining traction as a donor site for microsurgical reconstruction. In 2007, Ahmadzadeh and colleagues[11] conducted a cadaver study revealing that the profunda femoris artery gave off cutaneous perforators with large calibers, which could supply a significant portion of the posteromedial thigh. This laid the groundwork for the use of large PAP flaps in breast reconstruction, as described by Allen and Haddock[12] in 2012. The free posteromedial thigh flap was then reintroduced for head and neck reconstruction through a case series of 23 patients by Scaglioni and colleagues[13] in 2015.

The initial exploration of PAP flaps in head and neck reconstruction by Scaglioni and colleagues[13] marked a pivotal moment, providing a thorough examination of the anatomy, surgical methodology, and clinical applicability in 23 diverse facial, oral, and neck reconstructions. In the same year, Wu and colleagues[14] conducted the first comparative study between PAP flaps and ALT flaps, revealing PAP flaps' distinct advantages in terms of higher number of perforators (averaging 2) compared to ALT flaps (averaging 1.5) and the ability to close the donor site primarily, in contrast to ALT flap donor site necessitating skin grafts in some instances. This resulted in an ensuing surge in popularity of PAP flaps, yielding a multitude of landmark studies that explored surgical anatomy, techniques, and outcomes. In 2017, Fernandez–Riera et al.'s[15] detailed their experience with using PAP flaps to reconstruct 21 partial glossectomy defects, encountering only 2 minor complications, with favorable postoperative speech and deglutition assessments. In addition, Heredero and colleagues[16,17] explored important variants as the thin PAP flap and the chimeric PAP-gracilis flaps for glossectomy reconstructions, with one loss among the 10 thin PAP flaps due to vasospasm. Furthermore, Liu and colleagues[18] harnessed the pliability of PAP flaps to create individualized tongue models, reporting significantly superior speech, cosmesis, and deglutition outcomes compared to ALT flap reconstructions. Extending beyond oncologic applications, Loderer and colleagues[19] presented a case report showcasing the innovative use of PAP flaps in reconstructing progressive hemifacial atrophy, yielding favorable cosmesis albeit the need for subsequent thinning procedures. **Table 1** provides a comprehensive summary of all reports on free PAP flaps utilized in head and neck reconstruction over the past decade, encompassing data from over 360 patients.

Notably, our group has contributed some of the largest PAP flap studies to date in which we highlighted their reliability and consistent anatomy, even obviating the need for Doppler localization during vertical flap design.[6,20,21] The largest of these encompassed 61 PAP flaps, predominantly employed for tongue (n = 19), cheek (n = 11), parotid (n = 10), and maxilla (n = 6) reconstructions. Our flaps exhibited an average size of 7.1 × 12.1 × 1.9 cm, with a mean pedicle length of 11.5 cm.[21] Three partial flap losses occurred, and 8 patients required reoperation due to vascular compromise, hematomas, and infections. Seven patients experienced donor-site complications, with 2 necessitating operative intervention. In another study focusing on perforator mapping, we found the most common perforators to be A (33.7%) and B (33.7%), with B and C combined accounting for 18.1% only.[20] In a third study, we compared the ALT and PAP flaps in 65 subtotal and total glossectomy reconstructions. We found that in contrast to ALT flaps, PAP flaps were predominantly employed in patients with lower BMI, with comparable average flap volumes 7 months post-surgery. While swallowing/chewing and voice/speech were the most frequently reported high-severity items for both cohorts, patients reconstructed with a PAP flap demonstrated significantly improved swallowing function.

ANATOMY AND FLAP HARVEST
Profunda Artery Perforator(s) Anatomy

The PAP flap predominantly relies on perforators from the profunda femoris.[22] These perforators are known to emerge about 2 cm behind the gracilis muscle, approximately 8 cm below the groin crease.[23] In our clinical study mapping the vascular anatomy of 83 PAP flaps, we implemented a classification system akin to the one proposed by Yu and colleagues in 2004, categorizing perforators as A, B, or C based on their distance from the pubic tubercle.[20] The mean distances for A, B, and C perforators were 7.5 cm (range, 4–11.5 cm), 12.7 cm (range, 8–18 cm), and 17.6 cm (range, 14–20.5 cm) distal to the pubic tubercle along the adductor longus axis, and 7.9 cm (range, 6–12 cm), 7.3 cm (range, 5–12 cm), and 6.1 cm (range, 3.5–11.5 cm) posterior and perpendicular to the adductor longus axis, respectively (**Figs. 1** and **2**). Notably, A and B perforators predominantly exhibited large caliber, while C perforators were mostly of medium caliber. The musculocutaneous course was the most common for all 3 perforators, ranging from 84.6% to 97.8%. Two of our PAP flaps (2.4%) utilized separate pedicles for the same flap, while in 6.1% of cases, the A perforator originated

Table 1
Summary of free profunda artery perforator flaps for head and neck reconstruction in the past 10 years

Study	Number of Cases	Region(s)	Indication(s)	Reported Flap Length(s)	Reported Complications	Follow-up Range
Largo et al,[21] 2021	61	Multiple	Multiple	5–24 cm	• Recipient site: 10 major, 2 minor • Donor site: 2 major, 5 minor	0.2–30 mo
Ito et al,[24] 2016	48	Multiple	Multiple	8.5–32 cm	• 1 arterial thrombosis • 2 venous thrombosis • 3 partial necrosis	1–9 mo
Largo et al,[20] 2020	46	Multiple	Multiple	5–26 cm	• Arterial compromise • 8 donor-site dehiscence • 1 donor-site contour deformity	N/A
Chang,[41] 2023	35	• Oral • Maxillofacial • Neck	Multiple	Mean 9.8 cm	• 6 donor-site dehiscence • 1 fistula • 1 venous thrombosis	N/A
Ma et al,[49] 2022	33	Oral	Multiple	Average 12 cm	• 2 "flap crisis" • 2 wound dehiscence • 1 seroma	6 mo
Scaglioni et al,[13] 2015	23	• Oral • Face • Neck	Multiple	12–27 cm	• 1 flap loss • 1 flap infection • 1 flap dehiscence • 2 donor-site infections	2–7 mo
Fernandez-Riera et al,[15] 2017	21	Oral	Glossectomy (hemi)	N/A	• 1 hematoma • 1 prolonged intubation	~ 3 mo
Ismail et al,[36] 202	19	Oral	Glossectomy (total/subtotal)	10–16 cm	• 1 wound dehiscence • 2 infections • 1 hematoma • 1 partial flap necrosis • 3 delayed donor-site healing	7 mo
Wu et al,[14] 2016	18	• Oral • Maxillofacial	Multiple	N/A	• 1 hematoma • 1 partial flap loss • 1 wound dehiscence	3–8 mo

(continued on next page)

Table 1
(continued)

Study	Number of Cases	Region(s)	Indication(s)	Reported Flap Length(s)	Reported Complications	Follow-up Range
Kehrer et al,[50] 2018	12	• Oral • Maxillofacial	Multiple	10–26 cm	3 contractures	0–9 mo
Ciudad et al,[30] 2019	11	• Oral • Neck • Maxillofacial	Multiple	24–29 cm	• 2 donor-site (hypertrophic scar, permanent paresthesia)	Average 12.7 mo
Heredero et al,[17] 2020	10	Oral	Glossectomy (hemi/subtotal/total)	8–15 cm	• 2 infections • 1 wound dehiscence • 1 flap loss (vasospasm)	6 mo
Yao et al,[29] 2023	10	Face	Parotidectomy	N/A	N/A	8.1–19.5 mo
Iida et al,[48] 2019	7	• 4 Maxillofacial • 3 Neck	• 1 maxillectomy and 3 mandibulectomies • 1 hemiglossectomy, • 2 partial pharyngectomies	16–22 cm	Aspiration pneumonia	4–12 mo
Zheng et al,[60] 2022	3	• Orofacial	• 2 parotidectomy and neck dissection • 1 total glossectomy	12 and 18 cm	1 flap loss (vasospasm)	N/A
Liu et al,[22] 2023	3	• 2 Neck and Face • 1 Oral	• 2 parotidectomies + neck dissection • 1 glossectomy (total) + floor of mouth resection	12–18 cm	N/A	N/A
Mayo et al,[61] 2016	2	• Oral • Face	• Cancer resection • Gunshot wound	12 and 16 cm	None	N/A
Ramachandran et al,[53] 2023	2	Oral	• Buccal and floor of mouth resection • Glossectomy (partial)	15 and 22 cm	N/A	N/A
Loderer et al,[19] 2017	1	Face	• Progressive hemifacial atrophy	9 cm	None	13 mo
Karakawa et al,[54] 2020	1	Oral	(Hemi)glossectomy	18 cm	N/A	N/A
Heredero et al,[16] 2021	1	Oral	Glossectomy (total)	12 cm	N/A	2 year
Liu et al,[18] 2023	35	Oral	Glossectomy (hemi)	N/A	1 wound infection	12–32 mo

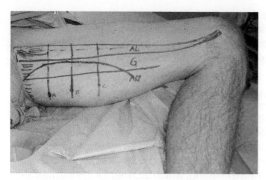

Fig. 1. The PAP flap harvest in frog-leg position with the preoperatively marked perforator location A, B, and C.

from the medial circumflex femoral artery rather than the profunda femoris artery. In 51 vertical PAP flap procedures, we found that 58.8% of the A, B, and C perforators merged during their courses, most commonly between B and C perforators (37.3%) and A and B perforators (17.6%). Lastly, while perforators A and B were identified in all 51 vertical flaps, 11.8% lacked a sizable perforator C. In 2016, Ito and colleagues[24] shared their experience with a smaller series of 48 PAP flaps. They identified a total of 95 sizable perforators, with the majority being musculocutaneous from the adductor magnus muscle (87.4%). The remaining 12.6% were septocutaneous, either between the adductor magnus and either the semimembranosus muscle or the gracilis muscle. The mean pedicle length stood at 9.8 cm. Among these 48 flaps, they encountered 3 cases of vascular thrombosis and 3 cases of partial flap necrosis, all of which were successfully salvaged. In the same year, Wu and colleagues[14] conducted the inaugural comparative study between PAP flaps and ALT flaps. PAP flaps exhibited a significantly higher number of perforators compared to ALT flaps,

with averages of 2 and 1.5, respectively. Despite this difference, both flaps demonstrated similar surface areas, dissection times, pedicle lengths, ischemia times, and complication rates. A distinctive advantage of PAP flaps was evident in donor-site closures, as all PAP flap sites could be closed primarily, whereas 3 cases involving ALT flaps necessitated skin grafts.

In a cadaveric study comparing upper thigh and buttock perforator flaps (including PAP, transverse myocutaneous gracilis, and fasciocutaneous infragluteal pedicles), Zaussinger and colleagues[25] showed that the PAP pedicle had the greatest mean external diameter and the second longest mean length in this region.

The Vertical Profunda Artery Perforator Flap Harvest

Key landmarks for the vertical PAP flap harvest include the gluteal fold, groin crease, posterior edge of iliotibial band, and the gracilis muscle. Classic techniques start harvesting from the upper third of the posterior thigh between the gluteal crease and the popliteal fossa. In our perforator mapping study, we described a reliable localization of the PAPs in frog-leg position for more accurate planning of the vertically oriented PAP flap without the need for imaging: flaps are primarily based on perforator A (33.7%) or perforator B (33.7%), with variations such as perforators B and C combined (18.1%), A and B combined (7.2%), perforator C (3.6%), and all 3 combined (1.2%).[20] However, we advise the use of a Doppler probe to confirm the mapped perforator location. A vertically oriented ellipse, encompassing the localized perforator(s), is carefully marked on the posteromedial thigh. Precise attention is essential during this process, as an anteriorly positioned incision in relation to the perforator location may compromise the flap width, posing challenges for primary closure of the donor site. This scenario is more common in individuals with minimal skin laxity, such as young patients and/or patients with obesity. Skin grafting for the PAP donor site is generally discouraged; therefore, if a skin graft is anticipated, an alternative flap should be considered for defect reconstruction. The subsequent harvesting of the flap occurs with the patient in the supine frog-leg or lithotomy position, facilitating an efficient 2 team surgical approach in head and neck reconstruction. The initial longitudinal incision, parallel to the gracilis muscle and following the marked flap design, extends through the gracilis muscle fascia into the subfascial plane until reaching the adductor magnus fascia. Following the fascial incision, the harvest progresses from anterior to posterior,

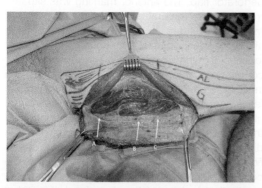

Fig. 2. The perforator A, B, and C location piercing through the adductor magnus muscle following subfascial dissection.

identifying the described PAPs. The selection of the most robust perforator is based on its location and size, typically requiring intramuscular dissection through the adductor magnus muscle to its origin from the profunda artery. Branches from the perforator supplying the adductor magnus muscle allow for inclusion of a muscular component with the flap if necessary. In cases where the pedicle delves into a voluminous adductor magnus muscle, the final dissection can be facilitated by creating an exposed window between the adductor longus and vastus medialis muscles. Postharvest, the flap is transferred to the recipient site following standard procedures, and the donor site is closed primarily in multiple layers, incorporating a closed suction drain for optimal wound management.

The Transverse Profunda Artery Perforator Flap Harvest

The transverse PAP flap yields a smaller skin paddle in contrast to vertical PAP flaps and is mostly based on the A perforator. The A perforator, however, has more variability in terms of location as described earlier. When harvesting a horizontal PAP flap, we advocate for the judicious utilization of preoperative computed tomographic (CT) angiography and/or preoperative or intraoperative Doppler ultrasonography.[26,27] This is underscored by findings from Cohen and colleagues[28], who observed that the majority of vertical PAP flaps had 2 perforators, versus only one perforator in most transverse PAP flaps.

Preoperatively, a transverse ellipse is meticulously marked on the patient in a standing position based on the A perforator. The superior border of this marking is positioned approximately 1 cm above the inferior gluteal crease. To determine the maximum flap width allowing for primary closure of the donor site, a pinch test is employed. We previously reported an average posteromedial thigh pinch of 4.6 cm, surpassing the 3.3 cm observed in the ALT.[20] Thereby, we recommend limiting the transverse skin harvest to 6 cm, in order to avoid imminent wound-healing issues. It is crucial to note that the flap design should not cross the gracilis muscle anteriorly nor should it cross the lateral border of the inferior gluteal crease posteriorly. The harvesting procedure can be conducted with the patient in either the lithotomy or supine frog-leg position. While a posteroanterior dissection is technically feasible, we recommend adopting the anteroposterior approach, as it enables the utilization of the descending branch of the inferior gluteal artery as an alternative vascular supply in case of perforator injury. An important consideration during this dissection is to remain in a suprafascial plane in order to preserve the posterior femoral cutaneous nerve and its branches, thereby preventing postoperative parasthesias along posteromedial thigh.

Alternative Flap Designs

In a study by Heredero and colleagues,[16] the feasibility of harvesting the PAP flap in a chimeric configuration, along with an innervated gracilis muscle, was explored. This approach was based on preoperative imaging, which allowed for the identification of the main gracilis pedicle's origin and its confluence with the PAP. Points where these perforators breached the deep fascia were noted, along with their relative positions from the ischium and the gracilis border. Flap elevation was executed above the deep fascia until the perforators were reached. Subsequently, the dissection continued through the adductor magnus and gracilis muscles, which included the main pedicle and the obturator nerve. The gracilis pedicle dissection was then extended until it merged with the PAP perforator(s) and eventually reached the profunda femoris artery. Nonetheless, this chimeric variant was only feasible in less than 30% of the study population, where a connection between the PAP and gracilis pedicle was identified through preoperative imaging. A variant of this flap was implemented by our group for facial reanimation and resurfacing, as will be highlighted later in this article.[29]

Ciudad and colleagues[30] demonstrated the viability of a transverse upper gracilis (TUG) perforator flap by integrating the TUG and PAP pedicles into a single, larger flap. Their surgical approach involved preoperative CT angiography and intraoperative Doppler mapping to assess perforator sizes, dominance, and pedicle locations. Notably, the preoperative identification of the TUG flap perforator held less significance as the TUG flap was harvested as a musculocutaneous flap rather than as a perforator flap. The anterior marking was situated medial to the femoral vessels, and the posterior marking extended to the midline of the thigh along the inferior gluteal fold, contingent upon the location of marked perforators. The superior border commenced anterolaterally, 1 to 2 cm below the inguinal crease, and curved in a semicircular fashion, maintaining a 1 cm inferior margin to the gluteal fold. The flap's width was determined through a skin pinching test, ensuring tension-free direct closures. Flap harvest starts in a plane superficial to the gracilis muscle fascia, extending to the posterior edge of the adductor longus muscle. A longitudinal incision of the deep fascia facilitated the identification and dissection of the gracilis vascular pedicle to its origin, preserving the greater saphenous vein. Superior and inferior transections of the gracilis muscle, in the desired length, facilitated suprafascial dissection for the PAP flap, approximately 3 cm posterior to the gracilis muscle. During flap elevation, the skin was undermined below the superficial fascia in an oblique fashion for larger volume flaps. The inclusion of gracilis not only adds substantial volume to the flap but also provides opportunity for restoring sensation through neurorrhaphy of the obturator nerve to recipient-site nerves, in addition to the possibility of a free functioning muscle transfer, as was reported by our group's experience with facial reanimation.[29]

Since PAP flaps were primarily designed for the purpose of breast reconstruction, the majority of its alternative designs were originally reported in this context. Nonetheless, we find no contraindication to employing these alternative designs in head and neck reconstructions if deemed necessary. One of these designs is the L-shaped PAP flaps, where our group strategically employed this design to achieve stacked PAP/lateral thigh perforator (LTP) flaps and bipedicled L-PAP flaps.[31] For the stacked PAP/LTP, a horizontal PAP flap was chosen along with an obliquely oriented LTP flap. On the other hand, the bipedicled posterolateral L-PAP flap was designed upon vascular territories of the upper medial, posterior, and lateral thigh, supported by the PAP and ascending branch of the lateral circumflex femoral vessels. This incorporated the pedicles of the PAP and LTP flaps, augmented by the inclusion of tissue in the midposterior thigh. The vertical PAP-upper gracilis flap, introduced by Skochdopole and colleagues,[32] encompasses vascular pedicles from both the medial circumflex femoral and profunda arteries perforators, maximizing the availability of medial thigh tissue in comparison to TUG flaps, PAP flaps, or the combination of both (ie, TUG-PAP). Another interesting design is the neurotized diagonal upper gracilis-PAP flap, originally introduced by Dayan and Allen.[33] The flap's design is bordered anteriorly by the posterior edge of the adductor longus muscle, curving posteriorly after a pinch test along Langer's lines. The posterior marking completed this ellipse, encompassing the PAPs. The flap was then neurotized via neurorrhaphy of the anterior obturator nerve with the lateral branch of the T4 intercostal nerve. However, neurotized flaps have not been used for head and neck reconstructions to date.

CLINICAL APPLICATION OF THE PAP FLAP IN HEAD AND NECK RECONSTRUCTION

Reconstructive strategies for head and neck soft-tissue defects hinge on various factors such as size, shape, depth, and location. In these cases, PAP flaps offer a myriad of advantages due to its ample volume, hairless skin, pliable fat content, consistent anatomy, reliable vascularity, and last but not the least, a hidden donor-site scar. In light of our expanding experience, we assert that this flap presents a versatile option for various microvascular reconstructions, shedding its historic status as a secondary option. In our study mapping the PAP flap vasculature, we consistently found at least 2 sizable perforators in every patient, complementing the angiographic findings by of DeLong and colleagues.[26] PAP flaps have also demonstrated superior cosmesis compared to ALT flaps, attributed to the posteromedial softer skin, more pliable adipose tissue, and hidden donor-site scar.[20] The PAP flap also stands out from a functional perspective due to its optimal thickness, making it an ideal choice for reconstructive procedures involving subtotal and total glossectomies, defects requiring maxillary sinus obliteration, or external cheek coverage, especially when adjuvant radiotherapy is anticipated. In general, in cases requiring additional volume, the adductor magnus muscle can be included, and flap orientation can be altered to various patterns, such as oblique, S-shaped, L-shaped, or even trilobed. Nevertheless, it can be argued that the inclusion of adductor magnus muscle with the PAP flaps reduces the pedicle length as the tissue components are connected more in series than in parallel as is the case with the chimeric ALT and vastus lateralis muscle flap. Beyond oncologic applications, Loderer and colleagues have showcased the innovative use of PAP flaps in reconstructing progressive hemifacial atrophy by de-epithelializing the flap.[19] Future studies should perhaps explore a "folded" variant of PAP flaps, where the flap is designed as 2 separate skin islands connected by deepithelialized skin, then folded on itself to simultaneously reconstruct external cheek and intraoral lining.[19]

While the ALT flap was historically the predominant workhorse choice, its inconsistent vascular anatomy occasionally prompts the use of an alternative option, such as the anteromedial thigh flap or a flap from the contralateral thigh.[14,34–39] In addition, ALT dissection often involves scarifying the lateral femoral cutaneous nerve, leading to paresthesias in up to 24% of patients.[40] In a comparative study involving 23 ALT flaps and 18 PAP flaps, both overall patient satisfaction and donor-site cosmesis perception were notably superior in the PAP flap group.[14] PAP flap is also superior to ALT flap in scenarios where pliability is crucial, particularly in tongue reconstructions. In these cases, the ALT is relatively rigid and frequently necessities chimeric configurations, such as the inclusion of the vastus lateralis muscle, which essentially atrophies upon adjuvant radiation, thereby leading to aspiration.

Nonetheless, cautionary measures are imperative when considering PAP flaps for patients with previous irradiation or surgery due to their shorter pedicle lengths that may necessitate vein grafts in this population. We approach the use of vein grafts with caution, limiting their deployment to situations of absolute necessity due to their associated high complication rate. In cases where a sensate flap is a requirement, the lateral femoral cutaneous nerve proves reliable and can be readily harvested with the ALT flap. In contrast, the PAP flap is typically insensate. It is also important to acknowledge the ergonomic challenges associated with PAP flap harvest in the frog-leg position. Additionally, incorporating multiple skin islands is more challenging with PAP flaps compared to ALT flaps, as PAP perforators tend to arise independently, while ALT perforators frequently converge on the main lateral descending circumflex femoral pedicle. As a practical recommendation, ALT flaps are suggested for cases requiring combined intraoral and extraoral components or situations necessitating chimerism.

Glossectomy Reconstruction

While traditionally considered an alternative in glossectomy reconstruction, the PAP flap has gained popularity due to its volume and pliability.[14,41] Given the PAP flap's notable pliability compared to traditional ALT flaps, this popularity has quickly grown over the past few years. Fernandez–Riera and colleagues[15] detailed their experience using PAP flaps to reconstruct partial glossectomy defects in 21 cases, encountering only 2 minor complications, with favorable postoperative speech and deglutition assessments. Heredero and colleagues[16,17] explored thin PAP and chimeric PAP-gracilis flaps for glossectomy reconstructions, with one loss among 10 thin PAP flaps due to vasospasm. Liu and colleagues[18] harnessed the pliability of PAP flaps to create individualized tongue models, reporting significantly superior speech, cosmesis, and deglutition outcomes compared to ALT flap reconstructions. In our recent study comparing PAP and ALT flaps for tongue reconstruction, we observed that PAP flaps are more feasible in patients with low BMI and provide significantly better deglutition, while no significant differences were noted in volume reduction or other functional outcomes.[6]

Subtotal and total glossectomies demand substantial tissue volumes, particularly due to sacrifice of floor-of-mouth muscles. Herein, the flap must be in contact with the palate in order to facilitate acceptable speech and swallow functions while minimizing the risk of aspiration. The flap's bulk also plays a crucial role in diverting saliva and food to the lateral gutters during swallowing, contributing to the overall goal of minimizing aspiration events. Notably, laryngeal suspension is an appropriate adjunct to reduce aspiration risk. This procedure involves compressing preepiglottic tissue and retroflexing the epiglottis, thereby closing the glottic opening during swallowing. Techniques for laryngeal suspension include suturing the posterior belly of the digastric muscle to the thyroid cartilage or suspending the hyoid bone, thyroid cartilage, or both, to the mandible.[42–44] Nonetheless, flap choice remains paramount, and a thick fasciocutaneous or myocutaneous flap is preferred. Drawing from our experience, the adductor magnus muscle can be included with the PAP flap, and flap orientation can be altered to varying patterns, such as oblique, S-shaped, L-shaped, or even trilobed, providing flexibility in reconstruction strategies. In addition, a chimeric gracilis-PAP flap can be harvested.[16] A comparative study conducted by our group evaluated PAP flaps against ALT flaps in subtotal and total glossectomy reconstructions, revealing no significant differences in donor and recipient-site complication rates or flap volumes at the end of a 7 month follow-up period (30.9% for ALT vs 28.1% for PAP; $P = .93$). Notably, patients who underwent reconstruction with a PAP flap demonstrated significantly improved swallowing function ($P = .034$).[6]

On the other hand, partial glossectomies requiring less flap volume can also be managed by PAP flaps. Heredero and colleagues described the thin PAP flap model that can be a good fit for this purpose. They customized the dissection plane based on patient needs and preoperative CT studies of the perforators. In their series, the depth of dissection could be made as superficial as above the superficial fascia layer.[16] The thin variant of the PAP flap is arguably preferred in partial glossectomy patients with low BMI, although less suitable for patients with higher BMI. In general, flap inset proceeds in a postero-anterior fashion, ideally preceding flap reperfusion, to enhance visualization. The sequence typically involves suturing the flap to the tongue dorsum first, elevating the posterior end of the flap. This approach prevents the drop-down of the tongue base and increases tissue volume on the posterior hemi-tongue, facilitating easier contact with the palate after reconstruction.

An intriguing innovation in tongue reconstruction with PAP flaps is the "Individualized and Convenient

Tongue Model" (ICTM) developed by Liu and colleagues.[18] Through analyzing the geometric anatomy of the tongue's surfaces, they created a paper model that considered the triangular shape of half of the tongue dorsum, the quadrilateral shape of one side of the tongue's belly, and the half-U shape of half of the tongue's floor. This model served as a layout for flap design using PAP or ALT, followed by flap raising and shaping by folding and suturing at previously marked spots. Liu and colleagues demonstrated the superiority of their ICTM model over conventional tongue reconstructions, showing significant improvements in speech ineligibility, swallowing, and cosmesis. The reported series indicated flap survival without donor-site complications, though one recipient-site wound infection occurred in the ICTM group. Furthermore, ICTM patients exhibited improved dietary intake, while conventional reconstruction patients experienced continued difficulties in drinking water, leading to a significantly lower quality of life in the conventional reconstruction group at the 12 month follow-up (85.68 ± 4.81 in conventional vs 104.89 ± 4.72 in ICTM, $P<.01$).

Parotidectomy Defect Reconstruction/Facial Reanimation

A radical parotidectomy, often involving facial nerve sacrifice, introduces considerable challenges to a patient's quality of life. The consequential soft tissue defect may lead to pronounced concave deformities that have been, historically, left unreconstructed. Additionally, facial nerve severance leaves patients unable to generate facial expressions or properly close their eyes. Reconstruction following radical parotidectomy becomes more complex when postoperative radiation or additional resections are required. Generally, the ALT flap is considered standard for volume correction and facial reanimation in these cases, particularly due to the availability of concomitant nerve and fascia grafts.[21,45] Nonetheless, the obturator nerve can also serve as a robust graft for facial nerve reconstruction in combination with PAP flap coverage. Notably, our group has modified the use of chimeric PAP flaps with functional gracilis to achieve adequate volume restoration and muscle function.[29] The gracilis muscle was accessed through a standard anterior incision, while the PAP flap was harvested through a separate posterior incision as previously described. At approximately 10 cm distal from the pubic symphysis, the neurovascular pedicle entering the gracilis was dissected and traced proximally. In cases where the gracilis pedicle converged with the PAP flap's pedicle, a chimeric

PAP-gracilis flap was harvested (3 of 10 patients); otherwise, the 2 flaps were harvested separately (7 of 10 patients). Innervation of the gracilis was achieved through multiple nerves, including the facial nerve stump, masseteric nerve, hypoglossal nerve, and spinal accessory nerve. Using this technique, dynamic reanimation with voluntary gracilis control was achieved in 6 of 10 patients, while the remaining 4 patients had a static sling to assist their speech and swallow functions.

Maxillectomy Soft Tissue Coverage

Maxillectomy poses a significant reconstructive challenge, given the functional and esthetic considerations in the midface. Beyond bony reconstruction, the importance of adequate soft-tissue coverage is paramount, particularly in larger defects where osteocutaneous flaps alone may fall short. In general, Brown classes 3 and above with involvement of cheeks and palate often demand free flap coverage, sometimes with multiple skin paddles.[46,47] This also holds true for other palatal or hemipalatal defects, irrespective of orbital floor preservation. The versatility of PAP flaps, with substantial soft-tissue volume, potential chimerism, and diverse orientations, makes them a reasonable choice in maxillectomy reconstructions.[20,21,30,41,48–50] However, it is important to remember that soft-tissue flaps alone can be complicated from intraoral ptosis, a challenge that may be addressed through suspension techniques and fascial incorporation.[51]

PITS AND PEARLS

The PAP flap has emerged as a valuable option in head and neck reconstruction, attributed to several advantages.[52] The robust and reliable PAP anatomy, often surpassing the ALT flap, showcases at least 2 sizable perforator in all PAP flaps. Our demonstrated technique leverages this anatomic advantage without necessitating preoperative or intraoperative imaging. We advocate for the use of a vertical orientation of the PAP flap in head and neck reconstruction to reduce donor-site complications. While the supine frog-leg position enables simultaneous harvest, its potential ergonomic discomfort should be acknowledged. Particularly beneficial for patients with cachectic head and neck cancer, the medial thigh provides substantial bulk when the ALT is insufficient.

Nonetheless, despite achieving an adequate pedicle length, surgeons should be cautious of the typically smaller pedicle artery diameter of the PAP flap compared to the ALT's descendant branch of the lateral circumflex vessels.[41] Further challenges arise in the limited experience with chimeric designs and alternative donor tissue options. The adductor magnus inclusion with the PAP flap may have restricted mobility compared to the ALT flap's vastus lateralis, but in specific circumstances, a chimeric gracilis PAP flap can be harvested. While multiple PAP perforators exist, they typically do not converge, complicating chimeric or double-skin paddle flap design. In cases especially requiring fascial autografts, for example, for static facial reanimation, alternate donor sites including the ALT might be more suitable.

Albeit the reliability of PAP flaps and the rare need for reoperation, developing strategies to manage technical failures in flap harvest is crucial. Thereby, Ramachandran and colleagues[53] introduced the concept of turbocharging PAP flaps as a salvage strategy in case of inadequate perfusion. In their case report, suboptimal perfusion to the flap resulted from eccentrically positioned PAPs, necessitating a perforator-to-perforator turbocharging technique. The side-branched stump was retained before clipping the distal perforator, and an end-to-end anastomosis was executed between the proximal perforator's stump and a branch of the distal perforator. The flap exhibited excellent vascularity without partial necrosis or complications 3 weeks postoperatively.

Some surgical refinements regarding lymphatic preservation and venous supercharging have also been suggested, albeit not being widely employed due to the rarity of relevant complications with PAP flaps. Karakawa and colleagues[54] found that the average distance from the medial femoral epicondyle to the intersection of collective lymphatic vessels and the anterior edge of the gracilis muscle was approximately 9.7 ± 1.6 cm, constituting approximately 30% of the total thigh length. To facilitate lymphatic preservation, they injected Indocyanine Green preoperatively and designed the PAP flap with borders that do not encompass any of these visualized lymphatic vessels. Intraoperative ICG visualization also guided the anterior dissection along the superficial fascia to avoid reaching the lymphatics. On the other hand, Iida and colleagues[48] used the posterior accessory saphenous vein, a branch of the great saphenous vein, as a lifeboat to supercharge PAP flaps complicated by venous congestion. This vein typically emerges at a location approximately 1 to 7 cm from the inguinal crease. The authors demonstrated sufficient venous drainage of the flap through the sole utilization of the posterior accessory saphenous vein.

In conclusion, the PAP flap emerges as a paramount choice for microvascular head and neck reconstructions, shedding its historic standing as a secondary alternative. With consistent identification of 2 sizable perforators in each patient and superior cosmesis compared to ALT flaps, it proves its versatility and reliability. The optimal thickness of the PAP flap makes it particularly advantageous in large defects and where adjuvant radiotherapy is anticipated. If additional volume is required with a PAP flap, the perforators relate to adductor magnus muscle for its potential inclusion and for possible flap reorientation into multiple patterns.[27,55] Studies have shown a 20% to 40% change in flap volume 6 to 12 months postsurgery, advocating for a 20% to 30% intraoperative overcorrection.[6,56–59] Furthermore, its adaptability extends beyond oncologic applications, as showcased in innovative reconstructions such as addressing progressive hemifacial atrophy. Overall, the PAP flap stands as a comprehensive solution offering both esthetic and functional benefits in diverse reconstructive scenarios.

CLINICS CARE POINTS

- PAP flaps offer ample volume, hairless skin, pliable adipose tissue, consistent and robust vascular anatomy, potential for chimerism, hidden donor-site scar, as well as straightforward harvest.

- The ample volume of PAP flaps is particularly beneficial for patients with cachectic head and neck cancer where other flaps may not provide sufficient volume.

- While various flap orientations are possible, vertical orientation is the most commonly used to mitigate donor-site complications.

- PAP flaps are ideal for voluminous defects, including defects following subtotal and total glossectomies, maxillectomy, and parotidectomy. Challenges with PAP flaps include a relatively small pedicle artery diameter and limited chimeric designs.

DISCLOSURE

No financial funding was obtained for this work. None of the authors has any conflicts of interest with any of the components of this work.

REFERENCES

1. Shuck J, Chang EI, Mericli AF, et al. Free lateral forearm flap in head and neck reconstruction: an attractive alternative to the radial forearm flap. Plast

Reconstr Surg 2020;146(4):446e–50e. https://doi.org/10.1097/PRS.0000000000007163.

2. Yu P, Chang EI, Selber JC, et al. Perforator patterns of the ulnar artery perforator flap. Plast Reconstr Surg 2012;129(1):213–20. https://doi.org/10.1097/PRS.0b013e3182362a9c.

3. Scaglioni MF, Meroni M, Fritsche E, et al. Superficial circumflex iliac artery perforator flap in advanced head and neck reconstruction: from simple to its chimeric patterns and clinical experience with 22 cases. Plast Reconstr Surg 2022;149(3):721–30. https://doi.org/10.1097/PRS.0000000000008878.

4. Contrera KJ, Hassan AM, Shuck JW, et al. Outcomes for 160 consecutive lateral arm free flaps for head and neck reconstruction. Otolaryngol Head Neck Surg 2023. https://doi.org/10.1002/ohn.596.

5. Agrawal G, Gupta A, Chaudhary V, et al. Medial sural artery perforator flap for head and neck reconstruction. Ann Maxillofac Surg 2018;8(1):61–5. https://doi.org/10.4103/ams.ams_137_17.

6. Ismail T, Padilla P, Kurlander DE, et al. Profunda artery perforator flap tongue reconstruction: an effective and safe alternative to the anterolateral thigh flap. Plast Reconstr Surg 2023. https://doi.org/10.1097/PRS.0000000000010890.

7. Conway H, Kraissl CJ. The plastic surgical closure of decubitus ulcers in patients with paraplegia. Surg Gynecol Obstet 1947;85(3):321–32.

8. Conway H, Griffith BH. Plastic surgery for closure of decubitus ulcers in patients with paraplegia; based on experience with 1,000 cases. Am J Surg 1956;91(6):946–75. https://doi.org/10.1016/0002-9610(56)90327-0.

9. Song YG, Chen GZ, Song YL. The free thigh flap: a new free flap concept based on the septocutaneous artery. Br J Plast Surg 1984;37(2):149–59.

10. Angrigiani C, Grilli D, Thorne CH. The adductor flap: a new method for transferring posterior and medial thigh skin. Plast Reconstr Surg 2001;107(7):1725–31. https://doi.org/10.1097/00006534-200106000-00013.

11. Ahmadzadeh R, Bergeron L, Tang M, et al. The posterior thigh perforator flap or profunda femoris artery perforator flap. Plast Reconstr Surg 2007;119(1):194–200. https://doi.org/10.1097/01.prs.0000244848.10434.5f.

12. Allen RJ, Haddock NT, Ahn CY, et al. Breast reconstruction with the profunda artery perforator flap. Plast Reconstr Surg 2012;129(1):16e–23e. https://doi.org/10.1097/PRS.0b013e3182363d9f.

13. Scaglioni MF, Kuo Y-R, Yang JC-S, et al. The posteromedial thigh flap for head and neck reconstruction: anatomical basis, surgical technique, and clinical applications. Plast Reconstr Surg 2015;136(2):363–75. https://doi.org/10.1097/PRS.0000000000001414.

14. Wu JC-W, Huang J-J, Tsao C-K, et al. Comparison of posteromedial thigh profunda artery perforator flap and anterolateral thigh perforator flap for head and neck reconstruction. Plast Reconstr Surg 2016;137(1):257–66. https://doi.org/10.1097/PRS.0000000000001880.

15. Fernández-Riera R, Hung S-Y, Wu JC-W, et al. Free profunda femoris artery perforator flap as a first-line choice of reconstruction for partial glossectomy defects. Head Neck 2017;39(4):737–43. https://doi.org/10.1002/hed.24675.

16. Heredero S, Falguera-Uceda MI, Sanjuan-Sanjuan A, et al. Chimeric profunda artery perforator - gracilis flap: A computed tomographic angiography study and case report. Microsurgery 2021;41(3):250–7. https://doi.org/10.1002/micr.30694.

17. Heredero S, Sanjuan A, Falguera MI, et al. The thin profunda femoral artery perforator flap for tongue reconstruction. Microsurgery 2020;40(2):117–24. https://doi.org/10.1002/micr.30485.

18. Liu M-D, Xue X-M, Al-Aroomi MA, et al. A novel flap design technique for subtotal tongue reconstruction with an "Individualized and Convenient Tongue Model". Oral Oncol 2023;145:106531. https://doi.org/10.1016/j.oraloncology.2023.106531.

19. Lóderer Z, Janovszky Á, Lázár P, et al. Surgical management of progressive hemifacial atrophy with de-epithelialized profunda artery perforator flap: a case report. J Oral Maxillofac Surg 2017;75(3):596–602. https://doi.org/10.1016/j.joms.2016.10.020.

20. Largo RD, Chu CK, Chang EI, et al. Perforator mapping of the profunda artery perforator flap: anatomy and clinical experience. Plast Reconstr Surg 2020;146(5):1135–45. https://doi.org/10.1097/PRS.0000000000007262.

21. Largo RD, Bhadkamkar MA, Asaad M, et al. The profunda artery perforator flap: A versatile option for head and neck reconstruction. Plast Reconstr Surg 2021;147(6):1401–12. https://doi.org/10.1097/PRS.0000000000007977.

22. Liu SW, Hanick AL, Meleca JB, et al. The profunda artery perforator flap for head and neck reconstruction. Am J Otolaryngol 2023;44(2):103772. https://doi.org/10.1016/j.amjoto.2022.103772.

23. Cormack GC, Lamberty BG. The blood supply of thigh skin. Plast Reconstr Surg 1985;75(3):342–54. https://doi.org/10.1097/00006534-198503000-00008.

24. Ito R, Huang J-J, Wu JC-W, et al. The versatility of profunda femoral artery perforator flap for oncological reconstruction after cancer resection-Clinical cases and review of literature. J Surg Oncol 2016;114(2):193–201. https://doi.org/10.1002/jso.24294.

25. Zaussinger M, Tinhofer IE, Hamscha U, et al. A head-to-head comparison of the vascular basis of the transverse myocutaneous gracilis, profunda artery perforator, and fasciocutaneous infragluteal flaps: an anatomical study. Plast Reconstr Surg 2019;143(2):381–90. https://doi.org/10.1097/PRS.0000000000005276.

26. DeLong MR, Hughes DB, Bond JE, et al. A detailed evaluation of the anatomical variations of the profunda artery perforator flap using computed tomographic angiograms. Plast Reconstr Surg 2014; 134(2):186e–92e. https://doi.org/10.1097/PRS.0000 000000000320.

27. Wong C, Nagarkar P, Teotia S, et al. The profunda artery perforator flap: investigating the perforasome using three-dimensional computed tomographic angiography. Plast Reconstr Surg 2015;136(5):915–9. https://doi.org/10.1097/PRS.0000000000001713.

28. Cohen Z, Azoury SC, Nelson JA, et al. The preferred design of the profunda artery perforator flap for autologous breast reconstruction: transverse or diagonal? Plast Reconstr Surg Glob Open 2023; 11(8):e5188. https://doi.org/10.1097/GOX.0000000 000005188.

29. Yao CMK, Jozaghi Y, Danker S, et al. The combined profunda artery perforator-gracilis flap for immediate facial reanimation and resurfacing of the radical parotidectomy defect. Microsurgery 2023;43(4):309–15. https://doi.org/10.1002/micr.30997.

30. Ciudad P, Huang TC-T, Manrique OJ, et al. Expanding the applications of the combined transverse upper gracilis and profunda artery perforator (TUGPAP) flap for extensive defects. Microsurgery 2019;39(4): 316–25. https://doi.org/10.1002/micr.30413.

31. Chu CK, Largo RD, Lee Z-H, et al. Introduction of the L-PAP flap: bipedicled, conjoined, and stacked thigh-based flaps for autologous breast reconstruction. Plast Reconstr Surg 2023;152(6):1005e–10e. https://doi.org/10.1097/PRS.0000000000010487.

32. Skochdopole AJ, Mentz JA, Gravina P, et al. Maximizing volume from the medial thigh: introducing the PUG flap. Plast Reconstr Surg 2021;148(2): 329e–31e. https://doi.org/10.1097/PRS.0000000000 008161.

33. Dayan JH, Allen RJ. Neurotized diagonal profunda artery perforator flaps for breast reconstruction. Plast Reconstr Surg Glob Open 2019;7(10):e2463. https://doi.org/10.1097/GOX.0000000000002463.

34. Yu P. Characteristics of the anterolateral thigh flap in a Western population and its application in head and neck reconstruction. Head Neck 2004;26(9): 759–69. https://doi.org/10.1002/hed.20050.

35. Shaw RJ, Batstone MD, Blackburn TK, et al. The anterolateral thigh flap in head and neck reconstruction: "pearls and pitfalls". Br J Oral Maxillofac Surg 2010; 48(1):5–10. https://doi.org/10.1016/j.bjoms.2009.07. 026.

36. Wei F, Jain V, Celik N, et al. Have we found an ideal soft-tissue flap? An experience with 672 anterolateral thigh flaps. Plast Reconstr Surg 2002;109(7): 2219–26. https://doi.org/10.1097/00006534-200206 000-00007. discussion 2227.

37. Celik N, Wei F-C, Lin C-H, et al. Technique and strategy in anterolateral thigh perforator flap surgery, based on an analysis of 15 complete and partial failures in 439 cases. Plast Reconstr Surg 2002;109(7): 2211–6. https://doi.org/10.1097/00006534-2002060 00-00005. discussion 2217.

38. Khadakban D, Kudpaje A, Thankappan K, et al. Reconstructive indications of anterolateral thigh free flaps in head and neck reconstruction. Craniomaxillofacial Trauma Reconstr 2016;9(1):40–5. https://doi.org/10.1055/s-0035-1558455.

39. Kimata Y, Uchiyama K, Ebihara S, et al. Anatomic variations and technical problems of the anterolateral thigh flap: a report of 74 cases. Plast Reconstr Surg 1998;102(5):1517–23. https://doi.org/10.1097/ 00006534-199810000-00026.

40. Collins J, Ayeni O, Thoma A. A systematic review of anterolateral thigh flap donor site morbidity. Can J Plast Surg 2012;20(1):17–23. https://doi.org/10.117 7/229255031202000103.

41. Chang EI. Alternate soft-tissue free flaps for head and neck reconstruction: the next generation of workhorse flaps. Plast Reconstr Surg 2023;152(1): 184–93. https://doi.org/10.1097/PRS.000000000001 0143.

42. Mok P, Woo P, Schaefer-Mojica J. Hypopharyngeal pharyngoplasty in the management of pharyngeal paralysis: a new procedure. Ann Otol Rhinol Laryngol 2003;112(10):844–52. https://doi.org/10.1177/ 000348940311201004.

43. Shin T, Tsuda K, Takagi S. Surgical treatment for dysphagia of neuromuscular origin. Folia Phoniatr Logop 1999;51(4–5):213–9. https://doi.org/10.1159/ 000021498.

44. Kos MP, David EFL, Aalders IJ, et al. Long-term results of laryngeal suspension and upper esophageal sphincter myotomy as treatment for life-threatening aspiration. Ann Otol Rhinol Laryngol 2008;117(8): 574–80. https://doi.org/10.1177/00034894081170 0804.

45. Fritz MA, Rolfes BN. Microvascular reconstruction of the parotidectomy defect. Otolaryngol Clin North Am 2016;49(2):447–57. https://doi.org/10.1016/j.otc. 2015.10.008.

46. Sakuraba M, Kimata Y, Ota Y, et al. Simple maxillary reconstruction using free tissue transfer and prostheses. Plast Reconstr Surg 2003;111(2):594–8. https:// doi.org/10.1097/01.PRS.0000041941.98504.B6. discussion 599.

47. Santamaria E, Cordeiro PG. Reconstruction of maxillectomy and midfacial defects with free tissue transfer. J Surg Oncol 2006;94(6):522–31. https:// doi.org/10.1002/jso.20490.

48. Iida T, Yoshimatsu H, Karakawa R, et al. Additional venous anastomosis in free profunda artery perforator flap transfer using the posterior accessory saphenous vein. J Plast Reconstr Aesthetic Surg 2019;72(12):1936–41. https://doi.org/10.1016/j.bjps. 2019.09.013.

49. Ma C, Gao W, Zhu D, et al. Profunda artery perforator flaps from the posteromedial region of the thigh for head and neck reconstruction. Otolaryngol Head Neck Surg 2023;168(3):345–56. https://doi.org/10.1177/01945998221109145.

50. Kehrer A, Hsu M-Y, Chen Y-T, et al. Simplified profunda artery perforator (PAP) flap design using power Doppler ultrasonography (PDU): A prospective study. Microsurgery 2018;38(5):512–23. https://doi.org/10.1002/micr.30266.

51. Sullivan M, Gaebler C, Beukelman D, et al. Impact of palatal prosthodontic intervention on communication performance of patients' maxillectomy defects: a multilevel outcome study. Head Neck 2002;24(6):530–8. https://doi.org/10.1002/hed.10095.

52. Chim H. Perforator mapping and clinical experience with the superthin profunda artery perforator flap for reconstruction in the upper and lower extremities. J Plast Reconstr Aesthetic Surg 2023;81:60–7. https://doi.org/10.1016/j.bjps.2023.01.001.

53. Ramachandran S, Chang C-W, Wang Y-C, et al. Turbocharging as a strategy to boost extended perforator flap vascularity in head and neck reconstruction-A report of two cases. Microsurgery 2023. https://doi.org/10.1002/micr.31111.

54. Karakawa R, Yoshimatsu H, Tanakura K, et al. An anatomical study of the lymph-collecting vessels of the medial thigh and clinical applications of lymphatic vessels preserving profunda femoris artery perforator (LpPAP) flap using pre- and intraoperative indocyanine green (ICG) lymphography. J Plast Reconstr Aesthetic Surg 2020;73(9):1768–74. https://doi.org/10.1016/j.bjps.2020.03.023.

55. Mohan AT, Zhu L, Sur YJ, et al. Application of posterior thigh three-dimensional profunda artery perforator perforasomes in refining next-generation flap designs: transverse, vertical, and s-shaped profunda artery perforator flaps. Plast Reconstr Surg 2017;139(4):834e–45e. https://doi.org/10.1097/PRS.0000000000003224.

56. Cho KJ, Joo YH, Sun DI, et al. Perioperative clinical factors affecting volume changes of reconstructed flaps in head and neck cancer patients: free versus regional flaps. Eur Arch Oto-Rhino-Laryngol 2011;268(7):1061–5. https://doi.org/10.1007/s00405-010-1450-5.

57. Yamaguchi K, Kimata Y, Onoda S, et al. Quantitative analysis of free flap volume changes in head and neck reconstruction. Head Neck 2012;34(10):1403–7. https://doi.org/10.1002/hed.21944.

58. Shin YS, Koh YW, Kim S-H, et al. Radiotherapy deteriorates postoperative functional outcome after partial glossectomy with free flap reconstruction. J Oral Maxillofac Surg 2012;70(1):216–20. https://doi.org/10.1016/j.joms.2011.04.014.

59. Tarsitano A, Battaglia S, Cipriani R, et al. Microvascular reconstruction of the tongue using a free anterolateral thigh flap: Three-dimensional evaluation of volume loss after radiotherapy. J Cranio-Maxillo-Fac Surg 2016;44(9):1287–91. https://doi.org/10.1016/j.jcms.2016.04.031.

60. Zheng L, Lv XM, Shi Y, et al. Use of free flaps with supermicrosurgery for oncological reconstruction of the maxillofacial region. Int J Oral Maxillofac Surg 2023;52(4):423–9. https://doi.org/10.1016/j.ijom.2022.04.019.

61. Mayo JL, Canizares O, Torabi R, et al. Expanding the applications of the profunda artery perforator flap. Plast Reconstr Surg 2016;137(2):663–9. https://doi.org/10.1097/01.prs.0000475776.22020.b6.

The Superficial Circumflex Iliac Artery Perforator Flap for Head and Neck Reconstruction

Mario F. Scaglioni, MD[a,b,*], Matteo Meroni, MD[a,b], Antonio Meschino, MSc[c,d], Gunesh P. Rajan, MD, DM, FRACS[e,f,g]

KEYWORDS

- SCIP flap • Perforator flap • Head and neck reconstruction • Microsurgery • Supermicrosurgery

KEY POINTS

- Head and neck defects present a unique challenge in reconstructive surgery due to the complex anatomy of this area.
- In the context of locally advanced head and neck malignancies, the established standard of care frequently involves the surgical excision of the primary tumor and concurrent neck dissection.
- The rectus abdominis musculocutaneous flap, anterolateral thigh flap, and radial forearm free flaps have commonly served as reliable choices for head and neck reconstruction.

BACKGROUND

In the context of locally advanced head and neck malignancies, the established standard of care frequently involves the surgical excision of the primary tumor and concurrent neck dissection.[1] Removal of malignancies in most cases involves making large tissue defects, which expose nasal and oropharyngeal cavities, neurovascular networks, thereby, increasing the risk of infection or hemorrhage. It is of high importance to address the resulting tissue defect through reconstruction with the goal to restore the typical oral and pharyngeal sealing while aiming for optimal functional and esthetic results with minimal complications.

In this setting, microvascular flaps emerge as the most appealing solution for the effective reconstruction of such defects. This is particularly noteworthy in specific head and neck locations such as the tongue or the floor of the mouth. The preservation of tissue mobility, pliability, and thinness is highly demanded to uphold overall functionality.

The rectus abdominis musculocutaneous flap, anterolateral thigh (ALT) flap, and radial forearm free flaps (RFFF) have commonly served as reliable choices for head and neck reconstruction.[2] However, it is crucial to acknowledge that the utilization of these flaps is followed by well-documented morbidity concerns. The ALT flap was considered as an alternative to the RFF flap due to a lower

[a] Department of Health Sciences and Medicine, University of Lucerne, Lucerne, Switzerland; [b] Zentrum für Plastische Chirurgie, Pyramid Clinic, Klinik Pyramide am See, Bellerivestrasse 34, Zürich 8034, Switzerland; [c] Faculty of Medicine of Vilnius University, Vilnius, Lithuania; [d] Dipartimento di Chirurgia, Ospedale Regionale di Locarno, Via all'Ospedale 1, Locarno 6600, Switzerland; [e] Department of Otolaryngology, ead & Neck Surgery, Luzerner Kantonsspital, Lucerne, Switzerland; [f] Otolaryngology, ead & Neck Surgery, Medical School, University of Western Australia, Perth, Australia; [g] Klinik für Hals-, Nasen-, Ohren- und Gesichtschirurgie, Luzerner Kantonsspital, Spitalstrasse 6000, Luzern 16
* Corresponding author. Zentrum für Plastische Chirurgie, Klinik Pyramide am See, Bellerivestrasse 34, Zürich 8034, Switzerland.
E-mail address: mario.scaglioni@gmail.com

Oral Maxillofacial Surg Clin N Am 36 (2024) 489–495
https://doi.org/10.1016/j.coms.2024.07.008
1042-3699/24/© 2024 Elsevier Inc. All rights reserved, including those for text and data mining, AI training, and similar technologies.

amount of morbidity. Some issues would still be present, such as the increased thickness of flap tissue when elevated from patients with high body mass index (BMI), large scars in exposed area, or a need for secondary debulking procedures to adapt the flap as a subsite for the soft palate or the tongue.[3]

A groin flap based on the superficial circumflex iliac artery (SCIA) was described for the first time by McGregor and Jackson in 1972[4] with a first successful application a year later by Daniel and Taylor.[5] This flap showed decreased harvesting morbidity as well as a more hidden donor scar. The popularity decreased due to a lacking variability of vascular anatomy, a short vascular pedicle, and the bulkiness of the flap demands meticulous fitting for optimal blood supply.[6]

The superficial circumflex iliac artery perforator (SCIP) free flap transfer has emerged as a promising technique in reconstructive surgery. This renewed advancement can be attributed to contributions by Koshima in 2004[7] and Hong in 2014,[8] whose landmark works introduced the SCIP flap. Their findings not only described the anatomic intricacies of the SCIP flap but also demonstrated the feasibility of elevating a thin flap with an extended and dependable pedicle. SCIP-free flap transfer offers several advantages in head and neck reconstruction. The donor site, located in the inguinal region, allows for inconspicuous scarring and minimal functional impairment. The reliability of the vascular pedicle minimizes the risk of flap compromise, making it suitable for complex reconstructions. The versatility of the SCIP flap extends its applications.[9]

The application of the SCIP flap for head and neck reconstruction has been minimally reported, but its ability to address defects in the oral cavity, oropharynx, and facial regions, coupled with ongoing advancements in surgical techniques, the SCIP flap emerges as a valuable and adaptable option, increasing the probability of success in reconstructive procedures within the complex landscape of head and neck surgery.[10–12]

ANATOMIC CONSIDERATIONS

The SCIP flap is supplied by perforator vessels originating from the SCIA, which also is responsible for the vascularization of the traditional groin flap. The SCIA emerges from the superficial femoral artery on its anterolateral aspect, about 3 cm below the inguinal ligament, and extends laterally, roughly 2 finger-widths beneath and parallel to the inguinal ligament.

The SCIA gives rise to 2 main branches. The superficial branch runs proximally over the sartorius muscle's fascia and distally into the fat tissue, producing several small-caliber perforators (0.3–0.5 mm) in the center of the anteromedial groin area. The deep branch instead lies under the deep fascia of the sartorius muscle, traveling in a superolateral direction and through the inguinal ligament. From an anatomic point of view, it is important to emphasize that typically, when the superficial branch is large, the deep branch tends to be shorter and thinner, while in some cases, where the deep branch is prominent, the superficial branch may be hypoplastic or even absent.

The venous outflow of the SCIP flap is supported by 2 primary systems located in the groin region, categorized as both superficial and deep. The superficial system is made up of the superficial circumflex iliac vein (SCIV) and the superficial inferior epigastric vein (SIEV), which are typically situated above Scarpa's fascia. Worth mentioning is that the SCIV and SIEV may merge medially to form a single larger vein ($\sim$2.5 mm in diameter), especially well-suited for anastomosis.

In certain cases, a segment of this common vein can be preserved together with the distal portion of the superficial iliac artery and utilized to lengthen the pedicle, especially in the perforator flap variant. The diameter of the SCIA typically surpasses 1 mm, but it can be smaller when a larger superficial inferior epigastric artery (SIEA) is present, which can partly supply the region.

SURGICAL PROCEDURE

From a technical point of view, we find that using the transverse branch as a guide for proximal-to-distal dissection the deep branch, following Yoshimatsu and colleagues's approach, is a useful approach that simplifies the harvest of the flap. This technique enables a complete dissection of the vessels, thus resulting in a longer pedicle.

We normally begin the dissection at the medial juncture, where the SCIA and SCIV emerge and join the superficial femoral artery and vein, respectively. To locate the vessels, we start with the incision on the medial edge of the flap area. These vessels' identification is crucial and precedes the final design of the skin island. Depending on the vessel orientation, adjustments to the flap's design can be made.

Typically, the primary perforator of the superficial and deep branches in the SCIA system is positioned at a juncture 3 cm medial to the anterior superior iliac spine (ASIS) along the SCIA pathway, thus the design of the flap should include this point and the region above the ASIS. In those cases where the pedicle is insufficient or absent, alternative vascular supplies such as the SIEA should be considered, or a shift to the contralateral side may be considered.

Closure of the donor site is achievable through direct suturing, although there are cases where a split-thickness skin graft may be required.

SUPERFICIAL CIRCUMFLEX ILIAC ARTERY PERFORATOR FLAP VARIATIONS

The SCIP flap is increasingly being recognized as a workhorse procedure in head and neck reconstruction especially because of its multiple variations. These comprise the possibility of harvesting very thin and pliable tissue in suprafascial plane or include other structures in a chimeric manner including bone, muscle, nerve, and lymphatic vessels.

Thin Flap

In its initial version, the traditional groin flap was characterized by a significant fatty layer, which cannot be safely reduced in thickness due to the axial pattern of the SCIA and its subfascial location on the medial side of the flap. However, with the advent of the groin perforator flap (SCIP), it is feasible to excise a substantial volume of fatty tissue with a careful resection around the perforator.[13] A suprafascial harvest is also possible, resulting in a very thin and pliable skin island particularly suitable for complex head and neck defect coverages (**Fig. 1**).

Osteocutaneous Flap

The superficial and deep branch can be also exploited to harvest a chimeric, multiple-tissue flap. This feature is particularly useful when bone tissue is also required. In our experience, we usually exploit the superficial branch to supply a thin skin island and the deep branch to vascularize the bone component (**Fig. 2**). As an alternative, the pedicle of the SCIP flap from the superficial circumflex iliac system can be anastomosed to the ascending branch of the deep circumflex iliac vessel. This combined osteocutaneous flap offers excellent blood circulation of the cutaneous portion. The iliac bone can be harvested based on the SCIA, but it is preferable to harvest it based on the deep circumflex iliac vessels.[14]

Muscle Flap

A segment of sartorius muscle can be harvested from the proximal portion of the SCIP flap if necessary. The inclusion of the sartorius muscle is determined by the presence of SCIA perforators that vascularize the muscle's upper segment. In instances where the SCIA penetrates through the

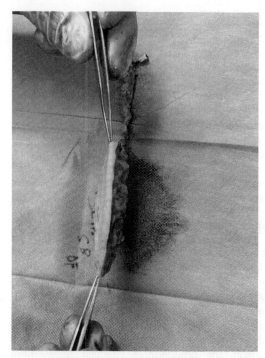

Fig. 1. Intraoperative picture of a thin suprafascial SCIP flap skin island at the end of the harvest procedure.

sartorius muscle, incorporating a portion of the muscle simplifies the elevation of the flap.[15]

Sensate Flap

Even if not frequently used, sensate flap variations are also possible. In 2011, Ida and colleagues described the use of the lateral cutaneous branches of the intercostal nerves for a sensate SCIP flap used for head and neck reconstructions. Another possibility resorts to the lateral femoral cutaneous nerve in order to form a sensate flap.[16]

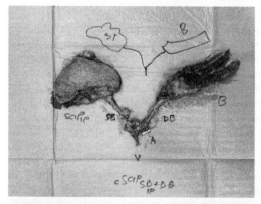

Fig. 2. Intraoperative picture of a chimeric SCIP flap including a bone component supplied by the deep branch and a soft tissue component supplied by the superficial branch.

Lymphatic Flap

The inguinal region offers a rich in lymphatic network that can be safely used for preventive lymphatic drainage restoration in the neck region. Recent advancements in the lymphatic field showed how the transplant of lymphatic vessels may have a significant impact in stimulating neolymphangiogenesis at damaged sites. This procedure, defined as vascularized lymphatic vessels transfer, has minimal donor-site morbidity compared to the well-known vascularized lymph node transfer and the SCIP flap is perfectly suitable for this kind of procedure.[17]

PREOPERATIVE ASSESSMENT

It is well recognized that the SCIA system presents significant anatomic variability in SCIP flap harvest and application. There are instances where the SCIA system can be hypoplastic or absent, requiring a different surgical approach. Hence, it is crucial to determine the dominant vascular supply in the flap's area before the surgery. For this reason, the preoperative vascular assessment represents a fundamental step when a SCIP flap-based reconstruction is planned. Recent advancements in the imaging greatly assist in this process. Different options are available for vascular mapping; our preoperative workup includes computed tomographic angiography (CTA) and hand-held Doppler mapping of the donor vessels. The latter is highly recommended because it is quick, simple, cost-effective, and easy to perform. It allows direct marking the vessel route on the skin (**Fig. 3**); however, a more comprehensive 3 dimensional visualization is achieved by combining Doppler findings with the results of CTA.

DISCUSSION

Head and neck defects have unique requirements and challenges that set this type of reconstruction procedures apart in the field of plastic surgery. The improvements of the medical and oncological therapies over the years lead to an increased number of patients, who are often old and fragile, elected for this kind of surgery, thus enhancing the perioperative and postoperative risks.

Achieving an ideal balance among soft tissue coverage, preservation of vital structures, and restoration of function is crucial in this area. Moreover, this area encompasses a wide variety of tissues. For example, the requirements for reconstructing the larynx or neck defects differ significantly from those for scalp reconstructions.[18]

Given the complex and delicate anatomy of the face, the principle of matching similar tissue may

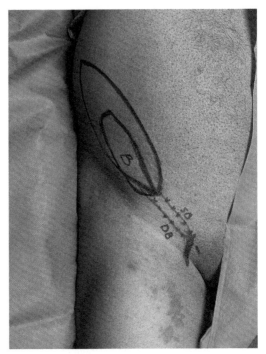

Fig. 3. Preoperative picture with skin markings showing the pathway of the superficial and deep branches. This planning is crucial before the harvest of chimeric SCIP variant.

require the simultaneous use of various types of tissue. In the maxillary region, in particular, bone defects are frequent, and they can be extensive, requiring large amounts of healthy bone and precise shaping for a successful result.

The SCIP flap is a very valuable tool for all these reasons. Once the limitations of anatomic variations are addressed, the advantages of the SCIP flap become evident. The tissues can be extensively customized in terms of shape, size, and thickness.[19] Additionally, various types of tissues can be harvested and arranged in a chimeric manner, including bone, skin, and fascia (**Fig. 4**).

The chimeric variation is a crucial feature that makes the SCIP flap so good for head and neck reconstructions, in particular when facing complex defects. This characteristic is extremely important, for example, in the case of tongue and oral reconstructions, or for hard palate and mandible reconstructions, or for extensive laryngeal and pharyngeal reconstructions.

In dealing with defects resulting from partial or hemiglossectomy, the SCIP flap is particularly suitable and presents a valid alternative to the more commonly used RFFF, which is associated with significantly higher morbidity (**Fig. 5**). The SCIP flap offers several advantages in this context. The skin paddle is usually thin, pliable, and capable of

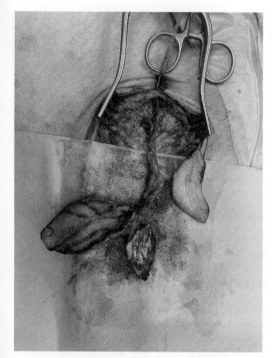

Fig. 4. Intraoperative picture of a multiple tissue chimeric flap including 2 separate skin island and a small portion of fascia.

excellent volume retention overtime. This characteristic is crucial for maintaining good functional outcome in the long term.[3] Other perforator-based options have been described for similar

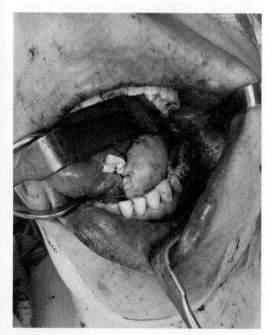

Fig. 5. The final result at immediate end of a lower left tongue reconstruction.

reconstructions, in particular the ALT flap. However, the groin tissue yielded better functional results when compared.[20]

The presence of 2 potential perforators with the superficial and deep branches introduces a higher degree of anatomic variability; however, at the same time, this feature offers an additional opportunity to sculpt the flap, as both perforators can be utilized to create a chimeric flap. Furthermore, once the main perforator is identified and chosen as flap's pedicle, its pathway to nourish the flap always runs in an axial direction and is relatively predictable. This allows for extensive thinning of the flap, even in patients with a high BMI.

Functional and sensory preservation is a notable postoperative advantage of SCIP flap procedures. The elevation of SCIP flap of standard variation does not require the dissection of muscles or nerves. This feature allows the retention of both functionality and sensory capabilities. Notably, there have been no reported instances of donor-site functional loss or sensorial disorders associated with SCIP flap elevation.[10] Alternative approaches such as RFFF elevation result in large donor-site morbidity and poor cosmetic outcomes, often requiring a skin graft for reconstruction.

From a technical standpoint, the perforator technique used in this flap allows for a shorter harvesting time and reduced donor-site morbidity. In the majority of cases, the donor site can be primarily closed, and it can be easily concealed, yielding good esthetic results.

Among the limitations of this flap, it is important to mention the possibility of encountering particularly small vessels that may require supermicrosurgical anastomosis with a diameter smaller than 1 mm. This technical difficulty is associated not only with the anastomosis process, but also with the dissection of the pedicle, which may be small and short in some cases. But such techniques as end-to-end or end-to-side anastomosis mostly using the superior thyroid artery seemed always possible according to literature published. Mostly requiring only one venous anastomosis.[10] A thorough and systematic preoperative vascular assessment is key step in preventing such complications. For this reason, in our practice, we always recommend combining CTA with hand-held Doppler evaluation and mapping.[21]

Intraoperative indocyanine green imaging has also become an essential examination tool for all our microsurgical procedures. We routinely use it during different stages of surgery to verify the perfusion of the flap before harvesting, after the anastomosis at the recipient site to assess the tissue margins' perfusion, and finally, at the end of the procedure, following the definitive inset (**Fig. 6**). This is

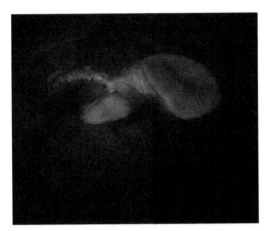

Fig. 6. Indocyanine green imaging under the microscope showing flap's vascularization at the end of the harvest procedure.

particularly valuable in this type of reconstruction, where the flap undergoes significant manipulation and is often positioned in unconventional orientations. Addressing these issues immediately during surgery can significantly contribute to reducing both partial and complete flap failures.[22]

SUMMARY

The SCIP flap represents an excellent reconstructive possibility for simple and complex head and neck defects. It provides pliable tissues that can be widely tailored according to the needs. Because of its peculiar anatomy, it can be also used in a chimeric manner, including multiple skin islands or different types of tissues, including bone, fascia, and muscle. All of this with a very low donor site morbidity, in body area which usually well tolerated by the patients. In our experience, all the reconstructive surgeons involved in head and neck surgeries should master this technique.

CLINICS CARE POINTS

- The SCIP flap is able to provide a large, thin, and pliable skin island that can be combined in chimeric manner with other tissues, including bone and muscle.
- The SCIP flap offers a wide range of tailoring in terms of extension and thickness of the transplanted tissues allowing to match the specific requirements of the recipient site.
- Recent advancements in terms of anatomic understanding of the inguinal region, combined with modern imaging techniques, allowed to

overcome the problem of the anatomic variation, historically related to the groin flap.

- The SCIP flap can be employed to reconstruct defects in the whole of head and neck region, including larynx, pharynx, intraoral lining, facial skin defect, or scalp defect.
- Supermicrosurgery is sometime necessary to dissect and to anastomose the smaller and shorter perforators. In these cases, smaller recipient vessels are necessary at recipient site for anastomosis.

DISCLOSURE

The authors have no financial conflicts nor commercial associations to disclose.

REFERENCES

1. Argiris A, Karamouzis MV, Raben D, et al. Head and neck cancer. Lancet 2008;371(9625):1695–709.
2. Disa JJ, Pusic AL, Hidalgo DH, et al. Simplifying Microvascular Head and Neck Reconstruction: A Rational Approach to Donor Site Selection. Ann Plast Surg 2001;47(4):385–9.
3. Ma C, Tian Z, Kalfarentzos E, et al. Superficial circumflex iliac artery perforator flap for tongue reconstruction. Oral Surg Oral Med Oral Pathol Oral Radiol 2016;121(4):373–80.
4. McGregor IA, Jackson IT. The groin flap. Plast Reconstr Surg 1973;52(2):217.
5. Daniel RK, Taylor GI. Distant transfer of an island flap by microvascular anastomoses. Plast Reconstr Surg 1973;52(2):111–7.
6. Hsu W-M, Chao W-N, Yang C, et al. Evolution of the Free Groin Flap: The Superficial Circumflex Iliac Artery Perforator Flap. Plast Reconstr Surg 2007; 119(5):1491–8.
7. Koshima I, Nanba Y, Tsutsui T, et al. Superficial Circumflex Iliac Artery Perforator Flap for Reconstruction of Limb Defects. Plast Reconstr Surg 2004;113(1):233–40.
8. Hong JP, Sun SH, Ben-Nakhi M. Modified superficial circumflex iliac artery perforator flap and supermicrosurgery technique for lower extremity reconstruction: a new approach for moderate-sized defects. Ann Plast Surg 2013;71(4):380–3.
9. Iida T, Mihara M, Yoshimatsu H, et al. Versatility of the superficial circumflex iliac artery perforator flap in head and neck reconstruction. Ann Plast Surg 2014;72(3):332–6.
10. Rosti A, Ammar A, Pignatti M, et al. SCIP flap in head and neck reconstruction after oncologic ablative surgery: a systematic review. Eur Arch Oto-Rhino-Laryngol 2023. https://doi.org/10.1007/s00405-023-08287-0.

11. Scaglioni MF, Meroni M, Fritsche E, et al. Superficial Circumflex Iliac Artery Perforator Flap in Advanced Head and Neck Reconstruction: From Simple to Its Chimeric Patterns and Clinical Experience with 22 Cases. Plast Reconstr Surg 2022;149(3):721–30.

12. Iida T, Yoshimatsu H, Yamamoto T, et al. A pilot study demonstrating the feasibility of supermicrosurgical end-to-side anastomosis onto large recipient vessels in head and neck reconstruction. J Plast Reconstr Aesthet Surg 2016;69(12):1662–8.

13. Park SY, Lee KT. Use of Super-thin Superficial Circumflex Iliac Artery Perforator Flap for Reconstruction of Lower Lip Defect. Plast Reconstr Surg 2023. https://doi.org/10.1097/PRS.0000000000010978.

14. Yoshimatsu H, Iida T, Yamamoto T, et al. Superficial Circumflex Iliac Artery-Based Iliac Bone Flap Transfer for Reconstruction of Bony Defects. J Reconstr Microsurg 2018;34(9):719–28.

15. Yoshimatsu H, Yamamoto T, Hayashi N, et al. Reconstruction of the ankle complex wound with a fabricated superficial circumflex iliac artery chimeric flap including the sartorius muscle: A case report. Microsurgery 2017;37(5):421–5.

16. Iida T, Yoshimatsu H, Hara H, et al. Reconstruction of large facial defects using a sensate superficial circumflex iliac perforator flap based on the lateral cutaneous branches of the intercostal nerves. Ann Plast Surg 2014;72(3):328–31.

17. Gentileschi S, Servillo M, Garganese G, et al. The lymphatic superficial circumflex iliac vessels deep branch perforator flap: A new preventive approach to lower limb lymphedema after groin dissection-preliminary evidence. Microsurgery 2017;37(6):564–73.

18. Wong CH, Wei FC. Microsurgical free flap in head and neck reconstruction. Head Neck 2010;32(9):1236–45.

19. Fernandez-Garrido M, Nunez-Villaveiran T, Zamora P, et al. The extended SCIP flap: An anatomical and clinical study of a new SCIP flap design [published correction appears in J Plast Reconstr Aesthet Surg. 2023 Jul;82:70]. J Plast Reconstr Aesthet Surg 2022;75(9):3217–25.

20. Watarai A, Yasunaga Y, Nakao J, et al. Groin and anterolateral thigh flaps for hemiglossectomy reconstruction: A comparison based on Japanese speech intelligibility. Auris Nasus Larynx 2023;50(1):110–8.

21. Yang JF, Wang BY, Zhao ZH, et al. Clinical applications of preoperative perforator planning using CT angiography in the anterolateral thigh perforator flap transplantation. Clin Radiol 2013;68(6):568–73.

22. Burnier P, Niddam J, Bosc R, et al. Indocyanine green applications in plastic surgery: A review of the literature. J Plast Reconstr Aesthet Surg 2017;70(6):814–27.

Pedicled and Perforator Flaps from the Facial and the Superficial Temporal Vessels

Laurent Ganry, MD, MSc[a],*, Beniamino Brunetti, MD, PhD[b]

KEYWORDS

- Head and neck perforator flaps • Head and neck pedicled flaps • Facial venous drainage
- Facial flap • Superficial temporalis flap • Head and neck reconstruction

KEY POINTS

- Local pedicled flaps based on facial and temporal superficial vessels are powerful tools typically used as a single-stage procedure for moderate-size facial defects.
- When a pedicled flap is designed to capture both arterial and venous vessels, the pedicle can be skeletonized with minimal risk of venous congestion.
- The venous system of the face is supported by a sizable venous loop composed of the facial vein, the supraorbital vein, and the frontal branch of the superficial temporal vein.

INTRODUCTION

Local pedicled flaps based on facial and temporal superficial vessels are powerful tools typically used as a single-stage procedure for moderate-size facial defects (smaller ones being treated with random flaps). They are incredibly convenient in areas with a higher risk of distortion (ears, eyes, nose, and lips) when there is a lack of skin laxity (younger patients) or in case of severe comorbidities (where free flaps may be more challenging).[1] Due to not uncommon anatomic variations in both systems, a preoperative Color Doppler or computed tomography scan with contrast is advisable preoperatively.[2] When a pedicled flap is designed to capture both arterial and venous vessels, the pedicle can be skeletonized with minimal risk of venous congestion. However, the venous pedicle can be far from its arterial pedicle in both systems. The facial vein is usually running posterior and lateral to the facial artery (up to 1–2.5 cm),

superior to the mandibular notch,[3] and the superficial temporal vein will always be found running close to its artery only in the preauricular area (but it is sometimes missing).[4] Harvesting a pedicled flap including these venous variations will lead to a higher flap success rate. Improving the flap's venous drainage is mandatory in all perforator variations of these pedicled flaps, as their designs will be done on an arterial pedicle. If designed on the facial/angular artery, a cuff of adipose tissue surrounding the perforator is highly recommended to increase venous drainage.

Furthermore, when a propeller perforator flap design is chosen, a reduction in complication rates is expected if a reduction of the rotational angle is planned.[5] If designed on the superficial temporal artery, it is essential to leave a large cuff of temporoparietal fascia (TPF) around the pedicle (up to a few centimeters if no vein can be identified) for the same purposes of increasing the venous drainage of the flap. In this scenario, large

[a] Department of Oral and Maxillofacial Surgery, Donald and Barbara Zucker School of Medicine, Long Island Jewish Medical Center, New Hyde Park, NY 11040, USA; [b] Plastic, Reconstructive and Aesthetic Surgery Department, Campus Bio-Medico University, Via Alvaro del Portillo 200, Rome 00128, Italy
* Corresponding author.
E-mail address: Laurent.ganry.md@gmail.com

Oral Maxillofacial Surg Clin N Am 36 (2024) 497–513
https://doi.org/10.1016/j.coms.2024.07.005
1042-3699/24/Published by Elsevier Inc.

incisions connecting the defect and the temporal donor sites are encouraged to avoid pedicle compression under subcutaneous tunnels and minimize the risk of venous insufficiency.

One could wonder how what seems to be a pedicled or a perforator flap design only on an arterial facial/angular or arterial temporal superficial system can still survive without any form of venous congestion, especially, when a vein is sometimes not visualized near the artery. Onishi and colleagues published complete facial venograms[6] highlighting a very dense network of small venous branches irradiating from the deeper subcutaneous vein (facial and superficial temporal vein) to the dermis, following the arterial perforators of the same arterial vessels (**Fig. 1**). Therefore, raising arterial perforators includes extremely small venous "perforators", not even visualized under microsurgical loops, which are drained into their distant large subcutaneous vein. This is why leaving a cuff of adipose tissue or fascia around the arterial pedicle in case of perforator flaps and some mucosal flaps is mandatory to increase a safe venous return in such locations.

The venous system of the face is supported by a sizable venous loop composed of the facial vein, the supraorbital vein, and the frontal branch of the superficial temporal vein. This loop presents very few venous valves and fuses with intracranial venous drainage at the medial canthus, allowing dual-direction venous drainage. Therefore, in both facial/angular and superficial temporal systems, reverse venous flow pedicle flaps present a low rate of venous congestion if designed correctly (such as a superiorly based nasolabial flap). Finally, the location with a higher risk of damaging the frontal branch of the facial nerve is when a flap is harvested on the infero-frontal branch of the superficial temporal artery (see later in the article[7]).

FACIAL/ANGULAR VESSELS PEDICLED FLAPS
Facial Artery Musculo-Mucosal Flap and its Island Version

It is a perfect example illustrating the risk of venous congestion depending on the flap design. The facial artery musculo-mucosal (FAMM) flap is an intra-oral arterial pedicle flap incorporating the facial artery, allowing the reconstruction of various mucosal defects in the ipsilateral oral cavity (superiorly or inferiorly based). However, to avoid venous congestion, the flap should never be islanded solely on the facial artery but instead left attached at its base to preserve a random submucosal venous drainage.[8] The pedicle is then divided during a second stage procedure (after its neovascularization). Despite this careful strategy, numerous FAMM flaps will become slightly venous to frankly congested (**Fig. 2**).

When the flap design includes the facial vein, the facial pedicle can be skeletonized until its origin in the neck, with minimum risk of venous congestion.[9] The flap's arch of rotation becomes wide. It bypasses the dental arch, making it possible to insert the flap by the neck directly through the floor

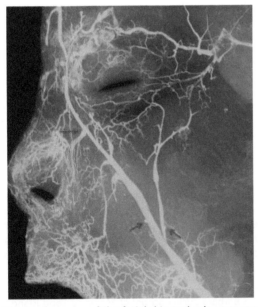

Fig. 1. Venogram of the facial skin and subcutaneous tissue. Venous valves (*red arrows*) are present in the polygonal venous network, but there are very few valves in the loop vein. (*From* S Onishi, N Imanishi, Y Yoshimura, Y Inoue, Y Sakamoto, H Chang, T Okumoto. Venous drainage of the face. J Plast Reconstr Aesthet Surg. 2017 Apr;70(4):433-440.)

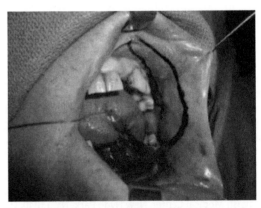

Fig. 2. Facial artery musculo-mucosal (FAMM) flap, designed with a large base and a 1.5 cm width centered on the facial artery. (*From* Ayad T, Xie L. Facial artery musculomucosal flap in head and neck reconstruction: A systematic review. Head Neck. 2015 Sep;37(9):1375-86.)

of the mouth or into the hypo- or oropharynx, offering a unique type of mucosal reconstruction in a single-stage procedure (**Fig. 3**).

Nasolabial Flaps

Nasolabial flaps are handy for understanding the concept of reverse venous flow and are powerful tools regarding ipsi and contralateral nasal and orbital reconstruction. They are a solid alternative to classic head and neck locoregional flaps, such as the paramedian forehead flap, with the benefit of being a possible single-stage procedure in selected scenarios. Typically, they can be selected when a paramedian forehead flap is inappropriate or could lead to significant complications or failure, such as for a patient who cannot undergo multiple procedures (severe comorbidities, unreliable patient), who is not concerned by the cosmetic outcomes, or with severe immunodepression (at risk of complications due to the paramedian flap exposed pedicle for few weeks).

These flaps can be designed on the facial artery or its most distal branch, the angular artery. The pedicle is usually superiorly based close to the medial canthus for a nasal or an orbital reconstruction or inferiorly based close to the alar crease in specific nasal reconstructions (see in the later section). The location of choice for facial vein ligation, separating a superiorly from an inferiorly pedicle-based flap, is usually realized at the cheek level, medial to the plan of the zygomatic muscles, along a vertical line passing by the V2 foramen (**Fig. 4**). This is because the facial vein becomes more superficial in this location and can be found running just deeper to the orbicularis oculi muscle. Usually, small V2 branches running superficially to the vein can be encountered.

When used to reconstruct multiple nasal subunits, a superiorly based nasolabial flap leads to more considerable nasal cutaneous tissue sacrifice (typically the lateral side of the nose), allowing a more cosmetic inset of the flap into the defect in a single-stage procedure (**Figs. 5** and **6**).

In 2 stages, more minor single nasal subunit defects can be treated with a lower superiorly based nasolabial flap as a perforator flap design (see in the later section).

An extreme arch of rotation can be developed to reach the contralateral side. The flap should always include the facial vein as a reverse flow venous drainage and be raised in the subperiosteal plan along the maxillary paranasal buttress to include the angular artery and its perforators (**Figs. 7** and **8**).

FACIAL ARTERY PERFORATOR FLAP
Rotational Perforator - "Plus" Flap

The melolabial flap is a powerful tool to reconstruct ipsilateral upper lip skin defects based on the perforators of the facial artery and vein, which are localized close to the modiolus region. The base of the flap is usually preserved, similarly to what is usually done with perforator-plus flaps (a combination of a pedicle flap including perforators in its design), to minimize scars and provide an additional source of venous drainage (**Fig. 9**). A huge

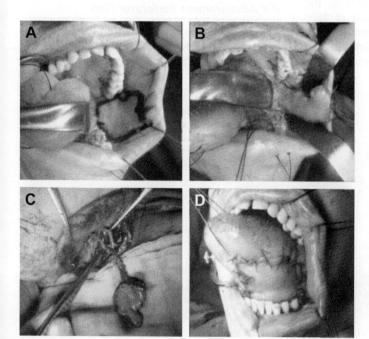

Fig. 3. Facial artery musculo-mucosal and its island version (FAMM-I) flap for the anterior and lateral floor of the mouth single-stage reconstruction in a non-edentulous patient. (*A*) Defect shape is reported on the cheek mucosa preserving Stensen's duct and oral commissure. (*B*) Facial artery and vein are isolated, ligated in the distal portion, and then dissected until their origin. (*C*) The flap is pulled out in the neck through a para-mandibular tunnel. (*D*) The flap is finally taken back inside the oral cavity through the floor of the mouth and then sutured to the recipient site. (*From* Vaira LA, Massarelli O, Gobbi R, Biglio A, De Riu G. Tactile recovery assessment with shortened Semmes-Weinstein monofilaments in patients with buccinator myomucosal flap oral cavity reconstructions. Oral Maxillofac Surg. 2018 Jun;22(2):151-156.)

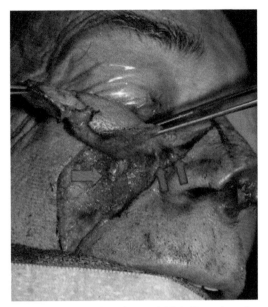

Fig. 4. Superiorly based nasolabial flap elevation, with visualization of the facial vein (*Blue arrowhead*) and the angular artery perforators (*Red arrowheads*).

donor site can be closed with a complementary cervicofacial advancement flap (Domino flaps) if necessary.

V-Y Advancement Perforator Flap

V-Y advancement flaps based on facial perforators are usually harvested in a random-pattern fashion similar to the melolabial rotational flap, usually for more minor defects. This time, the skin of the flap needs to be released at 360° from the surrounding tissue, and a central cuff of adipose tissue around the arterial perforators is maintained to preserve the flap vascularization

and facilitate venous drainage (**Fig. 10**). In case of a more extensive reconstruction or when an extended reach is required, the flap can be isolated on definite perforators, converting the flap into a pure facial artery perforator flap.[10]

Propeller Perforator Flap

Facial artery perforator propeller flaps are usually designed around 2 clusters of facial artery perforators: one located around the modiolus, expendable for upper lip reconstructions, and the other around the base of the nasal ala, chosen for lateral nasal reconstruction.[11] Once an explorative incision is performed to isolate the selected perforator, the flap is islanded, preserving the mimic musculature while maintaining a cuff of perivascular adipose tissue to facilitate venous drainage and rotated up to 180° to reach the defect without tension. The donor site is usually closed primarily (**Fig. 11**).

ANGULAR ARTERY PERFORATOR FLAP
Rotational Perforator-Plus Flap

A single subunit nasal defect, typically an alar defect, can be treated with a perforator-plus flap like a superiorly based lower nasolabial flap. However, due to the thin subcutaneous level of dissection associated with a close to 180° arch of rotation, it is safer to use this process as a 2-stage procedure. The base of the flap is left intact to increase the venous drainage of the flap, and the pedicle is divided into a second stage (**Fig. 12**).

V-Y Advancement Perforator Flap

As for a V-Y advancement flap on facial perforators, the V-Y advancement perforator flap on angular perforators comes with the same design

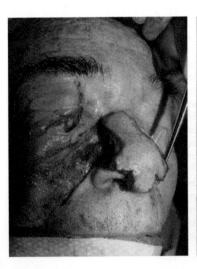
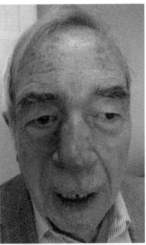

Fig. 5. Insertion of the superiorly based nasolabial flap for a tip/columellar defect in 1 stage procedure without further refinement. Note the minimum donor site morbidity without any ectropion.

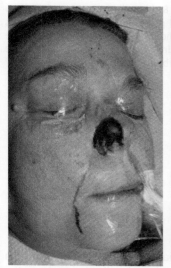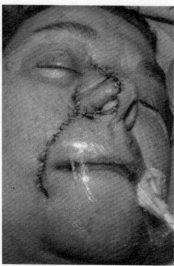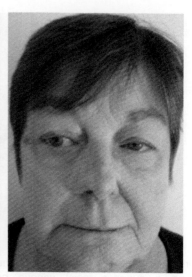

Fig. 6. Superiorly based nasolabial flap with concha cartilage graft for multiple nasal subunits reconstruction in 1 procedure without further refinement.

and execution. A more extended flap usually leads to better cosmetic outcomes (**Fig. 13**). Resection close to the lower eyelid/medial canthus[12] should lead to systematic flap suspension to the cartilaginous lateral nasal wall or the osseous lower orbital rim, preventing ectropion deformity. Suspension also helps to reduce the deformation of the flap secondary to lymphedema.

Propeller Perforator Flap

Angular artery perforator propeller flaps are usually employed with rotation less than 180° to reconstruct the ipsilateral nasal ala and nasal sidewall. The dissection is similar to the facial artery perforator propeller flaps, and the same surgical maneuvers are employed to reduce the risk of venous insufficiency (**Fig. 14**). The donor site is closed primarily along the nasolabial fold.[13]

COMBINATION OF BOTH WORLDS (FACIAL/ANGULAR PEDICLE)
Domino Flaps

A domino flap strategy can be performed when a superiorly based pedicled nasolabial flap on the angular artery and the facial vein is too wide to allow for primary donor site closure without causing an ipsilateral ectropion. To avoid this lower eyelid complication, a V-Y perforator facial advancement flap can be combined for primary closure (**Figs. 15** and **16**).

Bipedicle Flap

An interesting scenario is encountered when a lateral nasal defect sacrifices the angular artery but not the facial vein. In this case, a bipedicle nasolabial flap is possible, designed with an

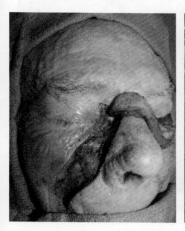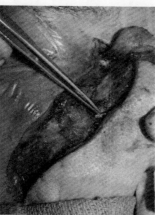

Fig. 7. Superiorly based nasolabial flap for contralateral orbital reconstruction in a single-stage procedure. The flap includes the facial vein and angular artery, and its dissection plane is below the periosteum on the paranasal maxillary buttress.

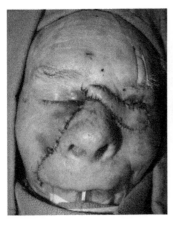 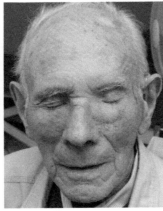

Fig. 8. Immediate postoperative photo and postoperative result at 6 months without further refinement. Note again the minimum donor site morbidity without any ectropion.

inferior arterial perforator close to the nasal base and a superior facial venous pedicle well-visualized during the dissection and included in the flap (**Figs. 17** and **18**).

SUPERFICIAL TEMPORAL ARTERY PEDICLED FLAP
Temporoparietal Fascia Flap

The TPF is a renowned flap to reconstruct cranio-facial defects. It is utilized in a pedicled fashion for the reconstruction of the scalp, auricle, facial soft tissue, orbit, oral cavity, and nasopharynx, as well as for skull base defects. However, it can also be pre-laminated for specific indications with a split-thickness skin graft (for intraoral lining, oro-cutaneous defect), pre-expanded (for facial burn defect – "Pie flap"[14]), or used as a free flap (laryngeal reconstruction, contralateral auricular reconstruction). There are a few essential critical

points during its harvest: the first is the meticulous plan of dissection when elevating the scalp, as the vessels are running relatively superficial in the TPF, just deeper to the thin layer of subcutaneous fat (**Fig. 19**). Second, the superficial temporal pedicle can be skeletonized only if a vein is visualized in the superior preauricular area. If a vein is not seen in the vicinity of the artery, a large cuff of 2 to 3 cm of fascia should be kept around the artery to maintain sufficient venous drainage. This last concept is the same for any superficial temporal artery perforator (STAP) flap harvested without clear visualization of venous drainage.

SUPERFICIAL TEMPORAL ARTERY PERFORATOR FLAP

A definite skin island harvested in the scalp or in the forehead regions and nourished by the terminal branches of the superficial temporal pedicle

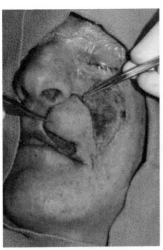 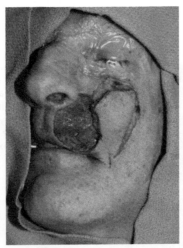 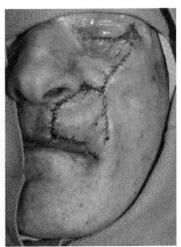

Fig. 9. Melolabial flap (facial artery perforator-plus flap) for upper lip reconstruction, based on facial artery perforators around the modiolus with a donor site close primarily without ectropion.

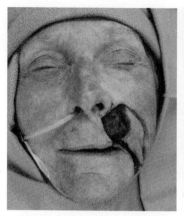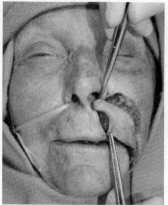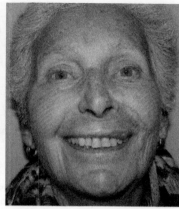

Fig. 10. V-Y advancement flap for smaller upper lip reconstruction, with a donor site close primarily. The postoperative result was at 6 months without further refinement.

defines the STAP flap, which is a peculiar cutaneous or fascio-cutaneous flap based on direct cutaneous vessels. Cranially to the zygomatic arch, the superficial temporal artery divides into 2 branches: the parietal branch (ascending vertically in the parietal scalp and sub-dividing in 2 terminal branches, named anterior and posterior, anastomosing with the occipital and the contralateral parietal vascular network) and the frontal branch (directed toward the forehead and sub-dividing in 3 terminal branches, named supero-frontal, centro-frontal, and infero-frontal, anastomosing with the ipsilateral and contralateral supratrochlear and supraorbital bundles) (**Fig. 20**).[7]

Any of these terminal branches can be used as a pedicle of a STAP flap, which can be harvested in the forehead for glabrous reconstructions of the periorbital region and midface, or an alternative in the scalp, for the hair-bearing reconstruction of the scalp, eyebrow, or sideburn.

Frontal Branch-Based Superficial Temporal Artery Perforator Flap

The frontal branch of the superficial temporal artery is an interesting donor site for locoregional glabrous flaps expendable for periorbital and midface defects. As stated earlier, the supero-frontal and centro-frontal branches should be used, and, if possible, the infero-frontal branch should be avoided. This arterial branch sometimes runs slightly inferiorly than usual, closer to the zygomatic arch and, therefore, nearer to the frontal branch of the facial nerve. This vascular variation places this arterial branch closer to the Pitanguy's line. The frontal branch of the facial nerve can even

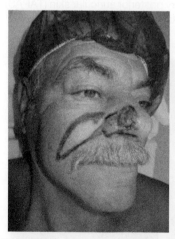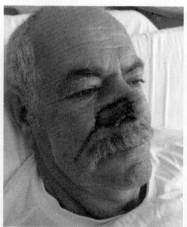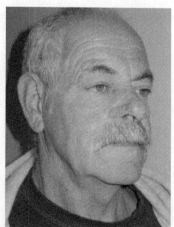

Fig. 11. Facial artery perforator propeller flap for 1-stage nasal ala reconstruction after basal cell carcinoma resection. Notice the transient venous insufficiency during the first 2 to 3 postoperative days. The postoperative result was at 6 months without further refinement.

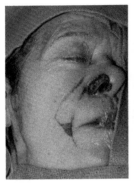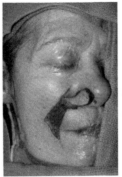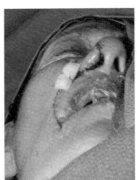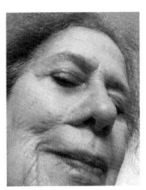

Fig. 12. Superiorly based perforator nasolabial flap with cartilage graft for single alar subunit defect in 2-stage procedure. Postoperative result at 6 months.

cross the vessel in some cases. However, the nerve would pass deeper to the vessel (and not superficially to it) in this location (the nerve will travel deeper into the superficial musculoaponeurotic system layer). Regardless, partial or complete forehead paralysis is possible if the flap is not raised close to the vessel's deeper aspect.[15] A thin skin flap can sometimes be harvested depending on the patient's tissues (from a glabrous thin forehead) with inconspicuous scars if taken at the junction with the hairline,[16] typically for more minor defects not exceeding 4 to 5 cm in width. Primary closure can be attempted if a brow-lift effect is desired (**Fig. 21**).

A laissez-faire technique can also be used for minor defects, allowing acceptable aesthetic outcomes on the forehead (**Figs. 22** and **23**).

Parietal Branch-Based Superficial Temporal Artery Perforator Flap

STAP flaps based on parietal branches help reconstruct scalp defects[17] or when replacement

of hair-bearing facial subunits (eyebrow, sideburn) is needed. Up to 3 to 4 cm of donor area defect can be closed primarily,[18] especially when designed in V-Y advancement, which gives an excellent advantage over skin grafting or artificial dermal matrice placement,[19] as split thickness skin graft can result in poor aesthetic outcomes secondary to skin color mismatch, thickness difference of the defect compared to the surrounding tissue, or alopecia.[20] Small STAP flaps are usually needed in case of sideburn or eyebrow reconstruction, allowing primary closure of the donor site and like-with-like reconstruction of the hair-bearing defect simultaneously (**Fig. 24**).

Parietal branch-based STAP flaps used for scalp reconstruction can be closed primarily for defects of 6 to 7 cm width when designed correctly (**Fig. 25**).

Temporal Artery Posterior Auricular Skin Flap

The temporal artery posterior auricular skin (TAPAS) flap, described by Lassus and colleagues,[21,22]

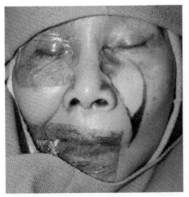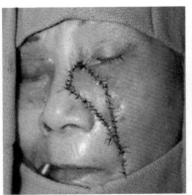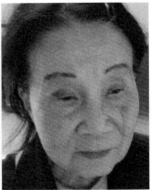

Fig. 13. V-Y advancement flap for smaller medial canthus reconstruction, with a donor site close primarily. Postoperative result at 3 months.

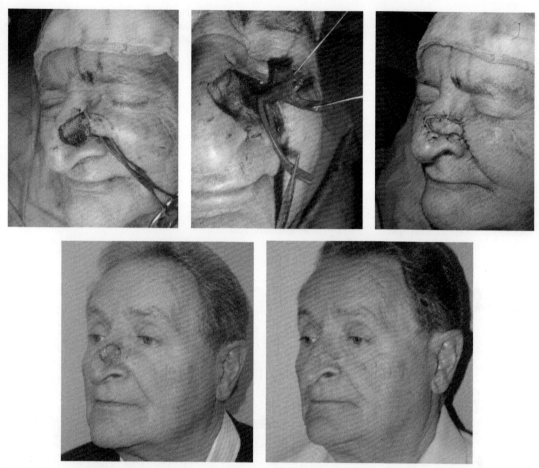

Fig. 14. 3 x 2 cm defect in the nasal sidewall after basal cell carcinoma resection in a patient refusing forehead flap reconstruction. An angular artery perforator propeller flap was harvested along the ipsilateral nasolabial fold and moved to the defect with a 120-degree clockwise rotation—preoperative and postoperative results at 6 months with a satisfactory outcome.

refined as a perforator flap by Ganry and colleagues,[23] is a thin cutaneous flap harvested from the glabrous posterior auricular region, and based on the superior auricular branch of the superficial temporal vessels. The TAPAS flap can be harvested as a 7 x 4 cm to 7 x 7 cm retro-auricular skin paddle (**Fig. 26**) to reconstruct multiple facial defects (**Fig. 27**). This perforator flap can be harvested with cartilage from the auricle (helix or concha area), and it is recommended to capture the

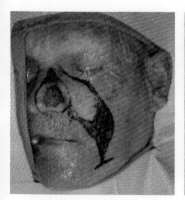

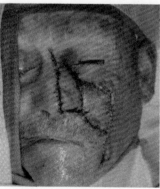

Fig. 15. Superiorly based wide pedicle nasolabial flap for hemi-nasal reconstruction without cartilage graft, combined with a V-Y perforator facial advancement flap in Domino Fashion to close the nasolabial flap donor site.

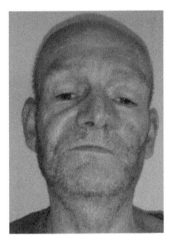
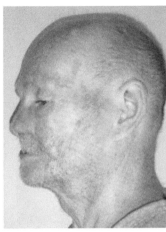

Fig. 16. Postoperative result at 1 year, without any refinements. Note the absence of ectropion.

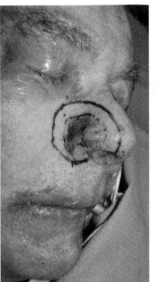
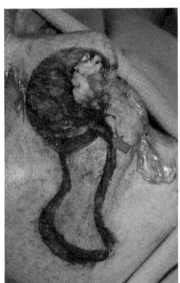
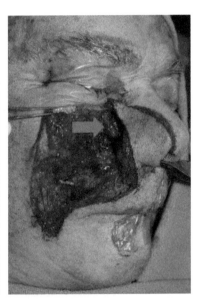

Fig. 17. Bipedicle nasolabial flap with cartilage graft in a single procedure, with visualization of the facial/angular artery perforators (*Red arrowheads*) and the facial vein (*Blue arrowhead*).

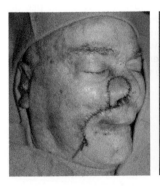
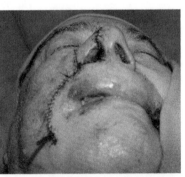

Fig. 18. Immediate result of a bipedicle nasolabial flap.

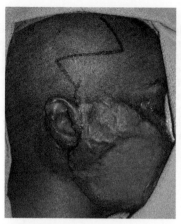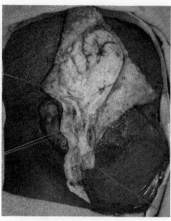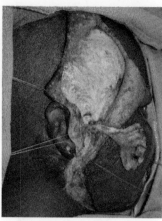

Fig. 19. First stage of a cervical "Pie flap" using a pre-expanded temporoparietal fascia (TPF) flap transfer in the neck to resurface in a second stage a significant ipsilateral cheek/midface post-burn sequel treated previously with multiple skin grafts.

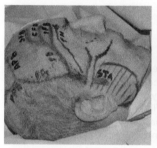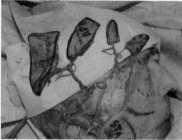

Fig. 20. Cadaveric dissection showing the terminal branches of the superficial temporal artery and the possible superficial temporal artery perforator (STAP) flaps to harvest in the fronto-temporal region. Notice the proximity of the anterior frontal branch of the facial nerve to the infero-frontal terminal branch of the superficial temporal artery (STA), limiting the use of this branch in the clinical practice to avoid forehead and eyebrow ptosis. (*From* Aveta A, Brunetti B, Tenna S, Segreto F, Persichetti P. Superficial temporal artery perforator flap: Anatomic study of number and reliability of distal branches of the superficial temporal artery and clinical applications in three cases. Microsurgery. 2017 Nov;37(8):924-929.)

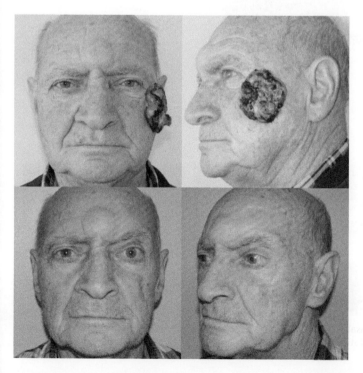

Fig. 21. Squamous cell carcinoma (SCC) resection in the zygomatico-temporal region with sacrifice of the frontal branch of the facial nerve. An 8 x 5 cm centro-frontal branch-based superficial temporal artery perforator (STAP) flap was used to reconstruct the defect with a rotational movement. The donor site was closed primarily to correct the expected brow ptosis. The patient is shown 6 months postoperatively with an excellent outcome.

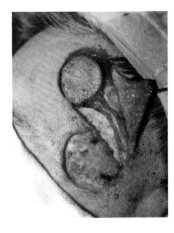
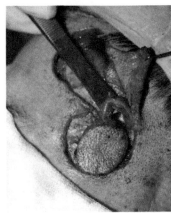

Fig. 22. Rotational centro-frontal branch-based perforator flap to reconstruct a minor superficial temporal defect preserving the frontal branch of the facial nerve, bringing glabrous tissue in a glabrous area. Note the meticulous development of different plans to preserve the nerve inferior and deeper to the pedicle.

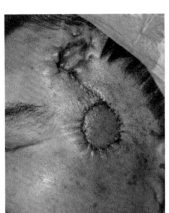
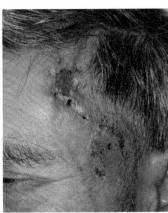

Fig. 23. Postoperative immediate and at 3 weeks results. Note the Laissez-faire healing of the donor site facilitated by a purse-string suture, as well as the flap's brief mild venous congestion (probably due to an excessive skeletonization of the artery).

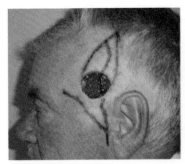
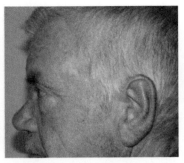
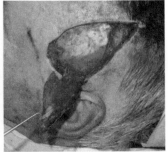

Fig. 24. Sideburn reconstruction after basal cell carcinoma (BCC) resection with parietal branch-based superficial temporal artery perforator (STAP) flap. Notice the complete restoration of an essential subunit for the male population in a like-like fashion.

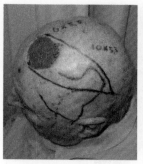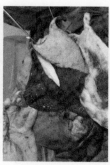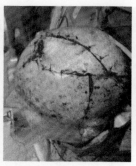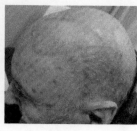

Fig. 25. Scalp reconstruction after basal cell carcinoma (BCC) resection (defect 6 x 5.5 cm) with parietal branch-based V-Y advancement superficial temporal artery perforator (STAP) flap (skin island 10 x 5.5 cm). Notice the wide fascial cuff surrounding the artery, which was spared to improve venous drainage. The donor site was closed primarily without skin grafts. The result shows complete restoration of the parietal scalp in a like-to-like fashion.

underlying fascia deeper to the subcutaneous fat to preserve a more robust venous return, such as in any flap using the superficial temporal pedicle.[23]

This perforator flap is an interesting reconstruction for a wide range of cutaneous facial small to middle-size defects (anterior auricular, temporal, orbital, nasal, and perioral) (**Figs. 28–32**) or as a free flap for intraoral, nasal, or intranasal septal defects. The donor site morbidity is minimal, allowing patients to wear glasses, ear aids, or facial masks for a few weeks after the surgery.

Preservation of a skin bridge inferior to the ear lobule is mandatory to allow for more robust venous drainage of the remaining auricle, and a simple primary closure is always sufficient even for a 7 x 7 cm defect (avoiding the use of skin graft, which could lead to severe ear deformities).

COMBINATION OF BOTH WORLDS (SUPERFICIAL TEMPORAL PEDICLE)
The Chimeric Temporal Artery Posterior Auricular Skin Flap

The TAPAS flap can be combined with multiple tissues, such as the pedicle TPF and all the

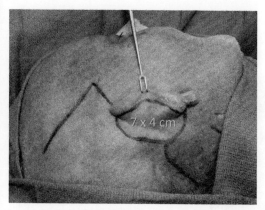

Fig. 26. Perforator TAPAS Flap classic donor site and size (up to 7 x 7 cm if needed). (*From* Ganry L, Ettinger KS, Rougier G, Qassemyar Q, Fernandes RP. Revisiting the temporal artery posterior auricular skin flap with an anatomical basis stepwise pedicle dissection for use in targeted facial subunit reconstruction. Head Neck. 2020 Nov;42(11):3153-3160.)

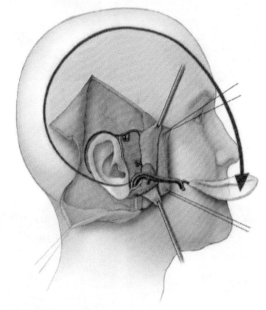

Fig. 27. Perforator temporal artery posterior auricular skin (TAPAS) flap maximum arc of rotation after extensive dissection of its superficial temporal pedicle into the parotid gland. (*From* Ganry L, Ettinger KS, Rougier G, Qassemyar Q, Fernandes RP. Revisiting the temporal artery posterior auricular skin flap with an anatomical basis stepwise pedicle dissection for use in targeted facial subunit reconstruction. Head Neck. 2020 Nov;42(11):3153-3160.)

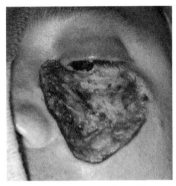 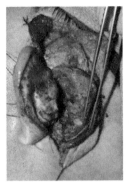 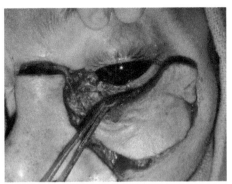

Fig. 28. 41-year-old male with a large midface defect post-resection of a basal cell carcinoma morphea type. Reconstruction with composite perforator temporal artery posterior auricular skin (TAPAS) flap, including a vascularized concha cartilage for lower eyelid and cheek reconstruction.

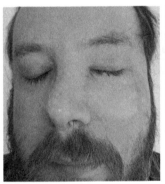 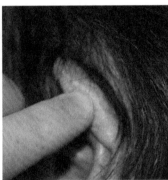

Fig. 29. Postoperative result at 1 year, without further refinement.

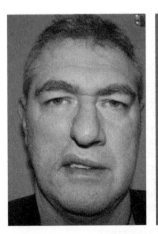 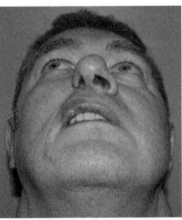

Fig. 30. 52-year-old male with a large upper lip and nose defect and retraction post-resection of a basal cell carcinoma (BCC) morphea type.

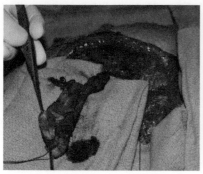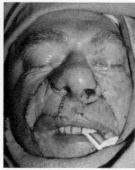

Fig. 31. Reconstruction with composite perforator temporal artery posterior auricular skin (TAPAS) flap, including a vascularized concha cartilage for nose and upper lip reconstruction.

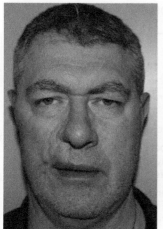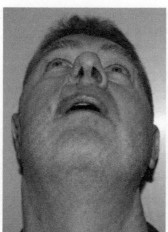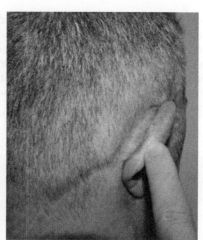

Fig. 32. Postoperative result at 1 year after a single debulking procedure.

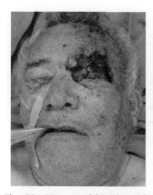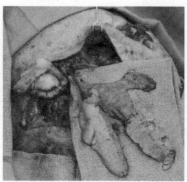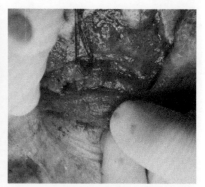

Fig. 33. 87-year-old male with a right functional eye presenting with a facial dog bite amputating his upper orbicularis oculi, upper eyelid, and eyebrow. Reconstruction with a pedicle chimeric temporal artery posterior auricular skin (TAPAS) flap combined with a temporoparietal fascia (TPF) flap supporting a hairy scalp skin paddle (eyebrow reconstruction) and a TPF layer (conjunctival layer reconstruction associated with a deeper buccal mucosal graft). The picture on the right demonstrates the insertion of the TPF paddle for the conjunctival layer reconstruction.

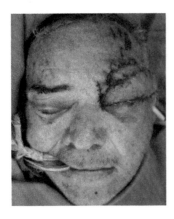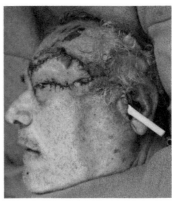

Fig. 34. Immediate postoperative result.

perforator flaps brought with it (including hair-bearing scalp, muscles, and even bone). Such designs using both the concept of pedicle and perforator flaps are powerful for reconstructing highly functional areas such as the orbital region, and the chimeric construct can stay pedicled in most cases (**Figs. 33–35**).

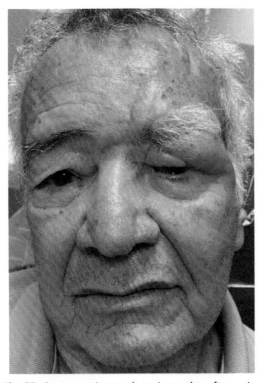

Fig. 35. Postoperative result at 4 months, after a single debulking procedure (upper eyelid and lateral aspect of the flap). Note the cosmetic outcomes and the balance obtained between eye protection and visual field amputation in a patient who has lost more than half of his superior orbicularis oculi.

CLINICS CARE POINTS

Pearls:

- These flaps are thin, pliable, and fast to be harvested but require meticulous soft tissue dissection.
- Vessel anatomic variations are possible.
- Facial and Superficial Temporal Flaps offer excellent like-by-like reconstruction for facial or intraoral defects.
- Facial vessels can harvest skin, facial hair, muscle, or mucosa, whereas temporal superficial vessels can harvest skin, hair, fascia, muscle, cartilage, or bone.

Pitfalls:

- These flaps can suffer from venous congestion.
- Superficial temporal pedicle flaps will typically not reach the nose or the central forehead regions.
- Avoiding complex pedicle dissection by converting a local superficial temporal flap into a free flap may be a faster and safer approach.
- Avoid these flaps in previously irradiated fields or if there were multiple surgical procedures in the area.

DISCLOSURE

The authors have nothing to disclose.

REFERENCES

1. Rougier G, Meningaud JP, Ganry L, et al. Oncological and aesthetic outcome following surgical

management of orbito-palpebral skin cancers: A retrospective study of 132 patients. Craniomaxillofac Surg 2019;47(10):1577–82.

2. Khorasanizadeh F, Delazar GO, Daneshpazhooh M, et al. Anatomic evaluation of the normal variants of the arteries of face using color Doppler ultrasonography: Implications for facial aesthetic procedures. J Cosmet Dermatol 2023;22(6):1844–51.

3. Cotofana S, Steinke A, Schlattau A, et al. The anatomy of the facial vein: implications for plastic, reconstructive, and aesthetic procedures. Plast Reconstr Surg 2017;139(6):1346–2135.

4. Imanishi N, Nakajima H, Minabe T, et al. Venous drainage architecture of the temporal and parietal regions: anatomy of the superficial temporal artery and vein. Plast Reconstr Surg 2002;109(7): 2197–203.

5. Brunetti B, Tenna S, Poccia I, et al. Propeller flaps with reduced rotational angles: clinical experience on 40 consecutive reconstructions performed at different anatomical sites. Ann Plast Surg 2017; 78(2):202–7.

6. Onishi S, Imanishi N, Yoshimura Y, et al. Venous drainage of the face. J Plast Reconstr Aesthetic Surg 2017;70(4):433–40.

7. Aveta A, Brunetti B, Tenna S, et al. Superficial temporal artery perforator flap: Anatomic study of number and reliability of distal branches of the superficial temporal artery and clinical applications in three cases. Microsurgery 2017;37(8):924–9.

8. Rahpeyma A, Khajehahmadi S, Sedigh HS. Facial artery myomucosal flap, pedicled solely on the facial artery: experimental design study on survival. J Craniofac Surg 2016;27(7):e614–5.

9. Vaira LA, Massarelli O, Gobbi R, et al. Tactile recovery assessment with shortened Semmes-Weinstein monofilaments in patients with buccinator myomucosal flap oral cavity reconstructions. Oral Maxillofac Surg 2018;22(2):151–6.

10. Hofer SO, Posch NA, Smit X. The facial artery perforator flap for reconstruction of perioral defects. Plast Reconstr Surg 2005;115(4):996–1003.

11. D'Arpa S, Cordova A, Pirrello R, et al. Reconstruction of nasal alar defects with freestyle facial artery perforator flaps. Facial Plast Surg 2014;30(3): 277–86.

12. Brunetti B, Tenna S, Aveta A, et al. Angular artery perforator flap for reconstruction of nasal sidewall and medial canthal defects. Plast Reconstr Surg 2012;130(4):627e–8e.

13. Lombardo GA, Tamburino S, Tracia L, et al. Lateral nasal artery perforator flaps: anatomic study and clinical applications. Arch Plast Surg 2016;43(1): 77–83.

14. Min P, Li J, Brunetti B, et al. Pre-expanded bipedicled visor flap: an ideal option for the reconstruction of upper and lower lip defects postburn in Asian males. Burns Trauma 2020;23(8):tkaa005.

15. Lei T, Xu DC, Gao JH, et al. Using the frontal branch of the superficial temporal artery as a landmark for locating the course of the temporal branch of the facial nerve during rhytidectomy: an anatomical study. Plast Reconstr Surg 2005;116(2):623–9.

16. Brunetti B, Tenna S, Poccia I, et al. Aesthetic reconstruction of the frontotemporal region: the extended a-t plasty, a workhorse revisited. Ann Plast Surg 2017;79(1):34–8.

17. Tenna S, Brunetti B, Aveta A, et al. Scalp reconstruction with superficial temporal artery island flap: clinical experience on 30 consecutive cases. J Plast Reconstr Aesthetic Surg 2013;66(5):660–6.

18. Algan S, Kara M, Cinal H, et al. The temporal artery island flap: a good reconstructive option for small to medium-sized facial defects. J Oral Maxillofac Surg 2018;76:894–9.

19. Brunetti B, Tenna S, Segreto F, et al. The use of acellular dermal matrix in reconstruction of complex scalp defects. Dermatol Surg 2011;37(4):527–9.

20. Dunham TV. A method for obtaining a skin-flap from the scalp and a permanent buried vascular pedicle for covering defects of the face. Ann Surg 1893;17: 677–9.

21. Lassus P, Lindford AJ. Free temporal artery posterior auricular skin (TAPAS) flap: A new option in facial and intra-oral reconstruction. Microsurgery 2017; 37(6):525–30.

22. Lassus P, Husso A, Vuola J, et al. More than just the helix: A series of free flaps from the ear. Microsurgery 2018;38(6):611–20.

23. Ganry L, Ettinger KS, Rougier G, et al. Revisiting the temporal artery posterior auricular skin flap with an anatomical basis stepwise pedicle dissection for use in targeted facial subunit reconstruction. Head Neck 2020;42(11):3153–60.

Designing Perforator Flaps Using Ultrasound

Alessandro Bianchi, MD[a], Akitatsu Hayashi, MD[b], Marzia Salgarello, MD[a],
Stefano Gentileschi, MD[a], Giuseppe Visconti, MD, PhD[a],*

KEYWORDS

- Ultrasound • Perforator flaps • High-frequency ultrasound • Ultrahigh-frequency ultrasound

KEY POINTS

- Ultrasound allows a detailed preoperative planning of flaps, providing topographic and dynamic information on the microanatomy.
- Ultrasound can be applied to tailor the flap thickness according to reconstructive needings based on individualized microanatomical information.
- Ultrasound is quintessential also in supermicrosurgical lymphatic surgery.

INTRODUCTION

The field of microsurgical reconstruction, as almost all the other surgical field, evolved together with the technological advancements, and so the introduction of the microsurgical instruments and techniques, the microscope, the progressive understanding of the vascular anatomy, and the imaging techniques.

Every step forward form the 80s to today, every achieved milestone, has in it the possibility of seeing what was invisible before, of predicting what was unpredictable before.

The perforators flaps are themselves an example of this revolution, because the difference from conventional to perforators flaps is only the ability to see smaller, and again smaller up the thin and superthin flaps, and even smaller up to the pure skin flaps, and free from limitations, up to the free-style flaps.

The Needing of the Preoperative Flap Planning

The early period of microsurgery was driven by the study of soft tissues microvascular anatomy, the understanding of the hemodynamics of flaps perfusion, and ultimately by the delineation of the vascular pedicles that allow to harvest the traditional fasciocutaneous, musculocutaneous, muscle and bony flaps.[1]

The traditional skin flaps are based on main vascular pedicles that, as major structures provided what proper names, are quite constant and maintain similar location and course in the human bodies, with few anatomic variations. The planning of these flaps was based on anatomic landmarks and, as the flap features are constant, they contributed to the affirmation of the concept of "flap of choice," in which a particular flap has the features that best match some reconstruction types.[2]

After the introduction of the angiosome concept by Taylor and Palmer in 80s,[3] and its clinical application by Koshima and Soeda,[4] the introduction of the perforator flaps changed the field of microsurgery. The following 20 years were focused on the discovery of new perforator flaps, and the applications of the most common perforator flaps in the clinical practice, with reports of outcomes and

[a] UOSD Chirurgia Plastica, Dipartimento Salute Donna, Bimbo e Sanità Pubblica, Università Cattolica del "Sacro Cuore" – Fondazione Policlinico Universitario "Agostino Gemelli" IRCSS, Largo A. Gemelli 8, Rome 00168, Italy; [b] Department of Breast Center, Kameda Medical Center, Kamogawa, Chiba, Japan
* Corresponding author.Largo Agostino Gemelli, 8, Roma 00169, Italy.
E-mail address: giuseppe.visconti@policlinicogemelli.it

Oral Maxillofacial Surg Clin N Am 36 (2024) 515–523
https://doi.org/10.1016/j.coms.2024.07.004
1042-3699/24/© 2024 Elsevier Inc. All rights are reserved, including those for text and data mining, AI training, and similar technologies.

indications to use. The increase in reconstructive options compared to traditional flaps affirmed the perforator flaps as a positive evolution, as they preserve muscle function, are less invasive, and able to accommodate the reconstructive needing, especially when the goal is resurfacing rather than creating volume and filling space.[1]

All these positive aspect are shadowed by the imperative knowledge of soft tissues and microvascular anatomy that cannot be approached with the intent of standardising that characterised the early microsurgical period.

The perforator flaps are based on smaller vessels, and as it comes to microanatomy, the anatomic variations are much more than traditional flaps.[5,6] The attempt to create the same system of reliable anatomic landmarks as for conventional flaps expressed through hundreds of anatomic works, with the creation of probabilistic x-y grids to help the surgeon to place his exploratory incision, and confirm intraoperatively the presence and the features of the perforator vessels.

But the microvascular anatomy of perforators varies from one patient to another, and there are areas in which perforators can take origin from different source vessels, such as the lateral thoracic area, the groin and the thigh. The intraoperative exploration is time consuming, more invasive, with a significant risk of failure, thus nullifying the major advances of perforators on conventional flaps.[7]

Moreover with the advent of Supermicrosurgery, pioneered by Koshima,[8] the ability to safely handle vascular structures below 0–8 mm represented a further expansion of the reconstructive freedom and a reduction in invasiveness. The possibility to harvest perforator flaps without dissecting the main vascular pedicle and the possibility of using perforating recipient vessels added another level of complexity.

Many levels of complexity have been added progressively, each one corresponding to an achievement in terms of freedom and reconstructive options.

The definition itself of perforator flap has been forced to change accordingly, from the first description based on the deep inferior epigastric artery perforator (DIEP) flap, of a skin flap without the deep fascia or the muscle based on a muscle perforator requiring intramuscular pedicle vessel dissection. The popularisation of anterolateral thigh (ALT) flap required the inclusion of septocutaneous perforators, so the definition changed to skin flaps based on vessels perforating the deep fascia, both muscle and septocutaneous vessels.[9] As the microanatomy was better known, the definition needed to include the chimeric flaps, such as perforator skin flaps with muscle or bone, and flaps without dissection of a pedicle perforating the deep fascia, like the superficial circumflex iliac artery perforator flap based on the superficial branch of the SCIA. In addition the flaps can be harvested at different vertical levels corresponding to different flaps thickness, depending of the branching features of each single vessel meant as pedicle.[10]

The modern concept of perforator flap is a target tissue elevated with the aim to selectively include a perforator perforating the corresponding envelope of the target tissue, whether it is the deep fascia for the muscle, the superficial fascia for the skin, the periosteum or the dermis.[9] But it is not only a matter of definition, it means to have at disposition all the 374 major perforators of the human body, and much more, to harvest a flap that suites the reconstructive needs. The dissection of a septocutaneous perforator is easier and faster than a musculocutaneous one, the elevation of a thin or superthin flap is safer, faster and more regular than a secondary thinning, the possibility to have an extra subcutaneous vein discharge can be a game changer, and other hundreds of examples could be presented.

The final concept is that microsurgeons have today the freedom of the "chosen flap," as opposed to the "flap of choice,"[2] but the preoperative knowledge of the microanatomy of each patient is mandatory.

The need for preoperative evaluation of the perforators, not only in terms of position, but also for dimensions, flow, and relationship with the surrounding structures became essential.

Imaging Modalities for Perforator Flaps

The imaging tools more commonly used in reconstructive surgery are Doppler ultrasound (hand held Doppler), computed tomography angiography (CTA), magnetic resonance angiography (MRA) and, ultimately, colour-coded Doppler sonography (CCDS).[7]

The Doppler sonography (hand held Doppler) was introduced in 70s and popularised in 90s for the perforator mapping.[11–13] It is used in several surgical specialities to locale and monitor vessels, and still represents the technology used by most microsurgeon to locate perforators and monitor the flap postoperatively. It is a portable unit, generally available in 8 and 10 MHz. Its diffusion is comprehensible if considering that is portable, cheap, easy to use, performable directly in the operating room and real time so the surgeon can mark the position of the signal on the skin. On the other hand this easy tool has many drawbacks, in fact the audible signal perceived by the unidirectional probe may correspond to any vascular flow, and it is impossible to distinguish a perforator from an indirect signal, a linking vessel, or the flow in a deeper structure.[14] The examination is influenced by variables such as the angularity and the pressure on the skin, so it is strictly operator dependent, but differently than CCDS, there is not a visual feedback that drives the operator. Above all, after locating a potential perforator, there is no information about the caliber, flow, corse, source vessel, relationship with the surrounding structures, and so the exploratory incision is still mandatory to confirm the findings and select the dominant perforator, and all the other variables can be revealed only during surgery, adding further complexity and potentially contributing to complication and failure.[14]

Because of all these limitations there was a great diffusion of CTA and MRA in preoperative perforator flap planning, probably with the attempt of limiting the operator-dependence of the examination and to delegate to radiologists the preoperative diagnostics.

The use of CTA has been largely diffused and it is part of the preoperative planning of DIEP flap of most microsurgeons. It is available in most centers, it allows for a rapid imaging of perforators and visualization of vessels up to 0–3 mm of diameter.[7] While Doppler ultrasound has the advantages of low cost and no radiation, the CTA showed to be obviously superior in locating perforators, in reducing the operative time and the rate of flap failure.[15,16] So the CTA became the examination of choice in many centers, and ultrasound in typically used to transpose the CTA findings on the skin. On the other hand CTA increases costs, require a complex organisation with a dedicated radiologist, it exposes the patient to radiation and requires intravenous iodinated contrast with risk of nephrotoxicity and severe allergic reactions.[6]

The MRA is preferred by some reconstructive surgeons due the radiation exposure and because the gadolinium-based contrast agent have minor probability of acute allergic reactions (0,07%) compared to CTA (3%). On the other hand the imaging takes a longer time, it costs more, is more prone to motion artifacts, and the smaller size of detectable vessels is 0,8 mm.[7,17,18]

Both CTA and MRA can provide clear anatomic images of perforator course though the muscle and the adipose tissue, bot technology cannot detect the exact size of perforators because the 2 examinations generally provide the image of the artery (enhanced by the contrast medium) while the vein remains not-enhanced. Moreover, both examinations are not real time and so do not allow a live marking of perforator location, that needs to be transposed on the patient skin by using a coordinate system o with the ultrasound examination.[13]

CCDS has been shown to have the highest sensitivity and positive predictive value to identify perforating vessels,[7] it is a powerful tool for preoperative perforator mapping in perforator flaps available to the plastic surgeon.[14,17,18]

It displays a real-time, color-encoded map of the blood vessels on the gray scale B-mode tissue image. The frequency of the probes commonly used in plastic surgery range from 4 to 19 MHz, the high-frequency ultrasound (>15 MHz) is useful to study the more superficial planes, so to focus on the distal portion of perforator vessels and superficial microanatomy.[1] The CCDS has a better spatial resolution than CTA and MRA, and high frequency probes allows a resolution up to 100 μm with the possibility of visualising microvessels up to 0,2 mm in size, that is a higher resolution than CTA and MRA. CCDS offers in depth and visual information about the size of perforators, the entire subcutaneous course up to the dermis, the flow velocity, and also about the tissues characteristics and the relationship with the sorrowing structures. The velocity scale and the color-code allows the evaluation of both perforator artery and comitantes venules. Due to the great diffusion of these technologies in many surgical and non-surgical field it is available in almost all centers, it costs less than CTA and MRA and, above all, it is a real time examination, that allow to modify the exploration focusing on the details needed in that particular reconstruction case, and allow to mark live the patient skin with high accuracy. This is particularly true not only because the examination is real time, but also because is performed in the same position of the patient as the operating room. The skin can be marked not only with perforator emergence, in fact by holding the probe in a longitudinal orientation is possible to determine the perforator axiality, and design the skin paddle accordingly.

The limited diffusion of CCDS is largely attributable to the learning curve,[6] and while many specialists have incorporated this technology in their daily practice, in plastic surgery it is not part of the training, even if CCDS represents the best technology to study the soft tissues and has many applications both in general plastic surgery and micro- and supermicro-surgery.

The latest evolution of ultrasound technology is the introduction of ultra-high frequency ultrasound. It involves the use of probes with frequencies as high as 48 and 70 MHz, with a correspondent resolution of 30 μm and 70 μm, respectively. It is possible to acquire unprecedented clear image of microscopic anatomic structures, with a detail level that is comparable to histologic examinations.[19–22] The main application of ultra high frequency ultraSound (UHFUS) is lymphatic surgery, but in some cases it can represent a useful tool for supermicrosurgical reconstruction. When it comes to blood vessels, the main limitation is the depth of penetration, that is 1 cm for the 70 MHz probe and 2 cm for the 48 MHz probe. For perforators UHFUS can be used as an adjunctive examination for the planning of thin, superthin and pure skin flaps, as it expands the knowledge of subcutaneous tissue anatomy and the microvascular network up to the tiniest branches and dermis entry point.[10]

Ultrasound-Guided Planning of Perforator Flaps

Among the literature about the use of ultrasound in reconstructive microsurgery, the preoperative mapping a perforators takes the largest part.[6] This is comprehensible because of all the advantages of this tool in detecting perforators and evaluating them along all their course, but it is also for the possibility of check the tissues and thus performing a virtual surgery that reduces the possibility of unexpected findings. Once the skill of ultrasound is acquired it is will be used also in the intra and postoperative period, in the selection of recipient vessels, and applied also to conventional non perforator flaps, as a fast tool to confirm the operative planning and avoid potential complications in almost all situations.

Conventional Perforator Flaps

The planning of perforator flaps is performed with the patient in the same position of the operating room, so to improve the accuracy of markings. In case of conventional perforator flaps, meaning the full thickness fasciocutaneous of adipocutaneous flaps, we use linear probes of 12 and 18 MHz.[14,19,21] (**Figs. 1 – 3**).

   At first the anatomy of the donor area is delineated by using the 12 MHz probe in B-mode. The examination starts from the deeper structure, like the muscles, bone, and the main pedicle. The main flap pedicle can be confirmed by switching to the color-coded duplex mode, and followed along its course up to the source vessel. At his point the gross anatomy is delineated, and the 18 MHz probe can be used for the identification of perforators by focusing on the muscle fascia. The traditional anatomic landmarks can be considered to begin the exploration, but all the donor is

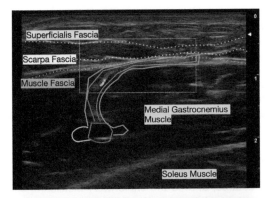

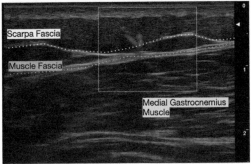

Fig. 1. Color-Coded Duplex Sonography of medial calf region to highlight the medial sural artery perforator flap vascular anatomy. (Above). The large red and blue circle represent the main pedicle (medial sural artery) within the substance of medial gastrocnemius muscle. According to the ultrasound study, we can trace the course of the perforator, which is a musculocutaneous perforator. Before piercing the muscular fascia, the perforator shows a 2 cm course just below the muscular fascia. (Below). The perforator has pierced the muscular fascia and we can start to appreciate its subcutaneous course. It is evident that the perforator starts to branch just above Scarpa fascia and this is classified as type 2 perforator.

systematically explored. The perforator is identified, followed along the course, the caliber and the flow can be measured. To follow the perforator down beyond the muscle fascia allow to determine if it is a musculocutaneous perforator, and in this case the length of the intramuscular course, or if it is a septocutaneous perforators. Generally the best perforator is selected according to caliber and flow and, when similar perforator are present, ultrasound (US) allows to choose the septocutaneous one that will have an easier dissection, or the one with an intramuscular course as shorter and less tortuous as possible. The perforators can be selected also according to their position in case of multiple skin paddles or in case of chimeric flaps, so to consider the pedicle length the allow flap insetting. The area surrounding the donor site can also be explored in case of non primary

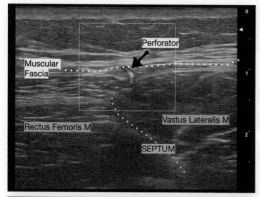

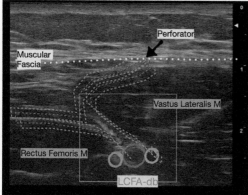

Fig. 2. Color-Coded Duplex Sonography of anterolateral thigh region to highlight the descending branch of lateral circumflex femoral artery (db-LCFA) perforator flap (also known as anterolateral thigh or ALT flap) vascular anatomy. (Above). The point where perforator pierces the muscular fascia is shown. (Below) According to the ultrasound study, we can trace the course of the perforator, which is located within intermuscular septum in its deep part and within the substance of vastus lateralis muscle in its more superficial portion before piercing muscular fascia. A muscular branch to rectus femoris muscle can be also traced.

closure, to locate perforators that can be eventually use to close the donor site.

Planning Thin, Superthin and Pure Skin Flaps

When thin, superthin or pure skin flaps are needed the US examinations is useful to clarify the microvascular anatomy of each perforator of each donor site, because in the same site it is possible to find perforators that fit or not a specific flap thickness, and choose the perforator accordingly to minimise the risk of failure.

We proposed in 2020 an ultrasound-based classification of thin perforator flaps and of suitable perforator.[10] High-frequency and UltraHigh Frequency probes allow to clearly define the subcutaneous anatomic planes, such as: subdermal,

Superficialis Fascia and Scarpa Fascia (**Fig. 4**). Those anatomic planes should be considered for harvesting anatomic thin flaps, as follows.

- Thin Flaps: flaps elevated along the Scarpa Fascia Plane;
- Superthin Flaps: flaps elevated along the Superficialis Fascia Plane;
- Pure-skin Perforator Flaps: flaps elevated along the subdermal plane.[5,6]

The perforators can be divided according to their arborisation in the subcutaneous tissue along they course, in 2 types.

- Type 1 perforator takes a direct course from the muscular fascia to the dermis, preserving their caliber until they reach the superficialis fascia, where they typically branch. Those branches clearly enter the dermis and connect to the dermal plexus vascular network. These microanatomical features make type 1 perforator adequate to harvest superthin or pure skin flaps, the dissection can proceeds along the selected plane of elevation up to the perforator entry point, avoiding the time for exploration or subsequent micro dissection of perforate branches. This approach reduces the risk of compromising the vascularity of the flap because the perforator has no relevant branches below the level of elevation.
- Type 2 perforators preserve their caliber from the muscular fascia to the Scarpa fascia, where they begin to arborize into collateral vessels within the subcutaneous tissue. Unlike type 1 perforators, type 2 perforators cannot be followed along their course from the muscular fascia to the dermis unless a tedious and dangerous microdissection with microscope is performed. This perforator type is adequate to harvest thin flaps, while should be avoided if thinner flaps are needed.

As previously mentioned, once a microsurgeon gets used to have all these information in its preoperative decision making, US will be applied in almost every field of reconstructive microsurgery, beside the design of perforator flaps.

We routinely use ultrasound to evaluate the recipient vessels in free-flap reconstruction, as it is possible to assess the needings of flap revascularisation such as the length of the pedicle, or eventually consider a perforator-to-perforator anastomoses.

Also for conventional non-perforator flaps the US examination can be useful, even if the anatomy and its potential variations are well known. US can

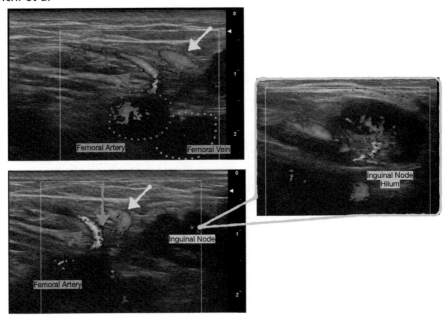

Fig. 3. Color-Coded Duplex Sonography of inguinal region to highlight the superficial circumflex iliac artery perforator (SCIP) flap vascular anatomy. (Above, left). Emergence of the superficial branch of the SCIP (red *arrow*) from femoral artery and vein. Just medial to the SCIP pedicle, the SCIV (superficial circumflex iliac vein) can be appreciated (blue *arrow*). (Below, left) The comitantes venule of the SCIP pedicle can be seen to enter the SCIV, and this information can be used to decide how to harvest the flap. On the right side, an inguinal node can be appreciated and this is important when inguinal lymphatic/lymph node flaps are harvested. (Right) Specific scans were done on the lympnode, highighting its hilum and also the vascular source that in this case is coming from SCIA and SCIV and not from superficial epigastric artery pedicle.

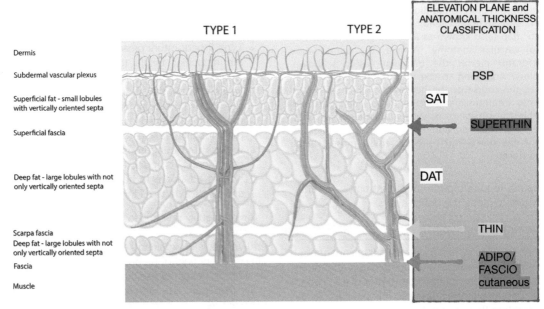

Fig. 4. Artist drawing of microvascular anatomy in the subcutaneous tissue. Type 1 perforator is a perforator that preserve its main structure up to the superficialis fascia where it can start to arborize or do directly toward the dermis. Those perforators are selected for harvesting superthin flaps (elevated on the plane of superficialis fascia) or pure-skin perforator flaps (elevated on the subdermal plane). Type 2 perforator is a perforator that usually arborize soon after piercing the muscular fascia, usually at the level of Scarpa fascia. Such perforators are not elegible for direct superthin or pure-skin perforator flaps unless microdissection is not performed. Type 2 perforator can be choosen for harvesting thin flap (direct elevation on the plane of Scarpa Fascia) or full-thickness adipocutaneous or fasciocutaneous perforator flaps. (with permission, *From:* Visconti G, Bianchi A, Hayashi A, Cina A, Maccauro G, Almadori G, Salgarello M. Thin and superthin perforator flap elevation based on preoperative planning with ultrahigh-frequency ultrasound. Arch Plast Surg. 2020 Jul;47(4):365-370. doi: 10.5999/aps.2019.01179. Epub 2020 Jul 15. PMID: 32718115; PMCID: PMC7398805)

be used to confirm the integrity of the vascular pedicle in a scarred area, or to locate the skin island of a myocutaneous flap including big perforators, so to increase safety, especially in complex reconstruction where the classic markings need to be modified according to peculiar reconstructive needings or previous surgeries.

PLANNING LYMPHATIC SURGERY

Ultrasound became quintessential in lymphatic surgery, either for supermicrosurgical lymphaticovenular anastomosis as well as for lymphatic flaps.

Ultrahigh-frequency ultrasound allows to expand knowledge of the very superficial anatomy, making lymphatic channels visible even when they are not detected by contrast-based technology such as ICG-lymphography.[22–32] Ultrasound allows to elucidate not only the presence of lymphatic channels, but also to define their number, size and their degeneration status with images comparable to the histologic examination. This helps not only in case of linear pattern after ICG-lymphography but also when no linear pattern are found,[26] ultrasound is able to find functioning lymphatic channels that otherwise are hided, thus allowing to expand indication for lymphaticovenular anastomosis (LVA) also to cases with no visible lymphatic channels at contrast-based examinations. Once lymphatic channels are found, ultrasound in then used to identify ideal recipient venules nearby, in terms of size, number of branches and no backflow.[30–32] In case no suitable recipient venules are find nearby the selected lymphatic channels, ultrasound allows alternative plannings as described elsewhere.

In lymphatic tissue transfer, ultrasound helps in understanding microvascular and lymphatic anatomy of the planned flap as for perforator and conventional flaps.

SUMMARY

Microsurgery has been continuously evolving in the last 40 years, and to make the most of all the increasing number of reconstructive possibilities and the consequent degrees of freedom, it is essential to have the exact knowledge of tissue and microvascular anatomy of each patient, that is peculiar and different from all the others.

Ultrasound technology has an higher sensitivity and specificity in perforator flap planning when compared with all the other technologies, and if performed directly by the operating surgeon represents the possibility of a virtual surgery before entering the operating room, thus improving safety, efficacy, reliability and, above all, creativity.

It represents the ultimate expression of the free-style flap concept, as it allows to choose the best perforator throughout the whole body that best fits the reconstructive needings in all aspects, including patient position, skin orientation, thickness needed, need for multiple skin paddle or chimeric configurations, matching with recipient vessels.

This technology is largely available, cheap, with no contrast injection, no radiation exposure, with the highest possible resolution, and time saving, as it eliminates the exploratory phase and the intraoperative decision-making.

We believe that ultrasound represents a true revolution in microsurgery and it has a great importance also in Supermicrosurgery, lymphatic surgery, and represents a support in many daily activities for all plastic surgeons.

CLINICS CARE POINTS

Pearls

- Portable and not-invasive technology
- Detailed preoperative knowledge of perforator location and course
- Detailed preoperative knowledge of perforator dynamics
- Detailed preoperative knowledge of perforator course in subcutaneous tissue for primary flap thinning
- Ultrasound allows postoperative monitoring of flaps
- Detailed preoperative knowledge of lymphatic and venule anatomy

Pitfall

- Needing to master this technology to be applied by the operating surgeon

DISCLOSURE

The authors have nothing to disclose.

REFERENCES

1. Visconti G, Hayashi A, Hong JP. The New Imaging Techniques in Reconstructive Microsurgery: A New Revolution in Perforator Flaps and Lymphatic Surgery. Arch Plast Surg 2022;49(4):471–2. https://doi.org/10.1055/s-0042-1751099.
2. Kim JT, Kim SW. Perforator Flap versus Conventional Flap. J Kor Med Sci 2015;30(5):514–22.

3. Taylor GI, Palmer JH. The vascular territories (angiosomes) of the body: experimental study and clinical applications. Br J Plast Surg 1987;40(02):113–41.

4. Koshima I, Soeda S. Inferior epigastric artery skin flaps without rectus abdominis muscle. Br J Plast Surg 1989;42(06):645–8.

5. Visconti G, Hayashi A, Yoshimatsu H, et al. Ultra-high frequency ultrasound in planning capillary perforator flaps: Preliminary experience. J Plast Reconstr Aesthetic Surg 2018;71(8):1146–52. https://doi.org/10.1016/j.bjps.2018.05.045.

6. Visconti G, Bianchi A, Hayashi A, et al. Pure skin perforator flap direct elevation above the subdermal plane using preoperative ultra-high frequency ultrasound planning: A proof of concept. J Plast Reconstr Aesthetic Surg 2019;72(10):1700–38.

7. Cho MJ, Kwon JG, Pak CJ, et al. The Role of Duplex Ultrasound in Microsurgical Reconstruction: Review and Technical Considerations. J Reconstr Microsurg 2020;36(7):514–21. https://doi.org/10.1055/s-0040-1709479.

8. Koshima I, Inagawa K, Etoh K, et al. [Supramicrosurgical lymphaticovenular anastomosis for the treatment of lymphede- ma in the extremities]. Nippon Geka Gakkai Zasshi 1999;100(09):551–6.

9. Yamamoto T, Yamamoto N, Kageyama T, et al. Definition of perforator flap: what does a "perforator" perforate? Glob Health Med 2019;1(2):114–6. https://doi.org/10.35772/ghm.2019.01009.

10. Visconti G, Bianchi A, Hayashi A, et al. Thin and superthin perforator flap elevation based on preoperative planning with ultrahigh-frequency ultrasound. Arch Plast Surg 2020;47(4):365–70. https://doi.org/10.5999/aps.2019.01179.

11. Aoyagi F, Fujino T, Ohshiro T. Detection of small vessels for microsurgery by a Doppler flowmeter. Plast Reconstr Surg 1975;55(3):372–3.

12. Karkowski J, Buncke HJ. A simplified technique for free transfer of groin flaps, by use of a Doppler probe. Plast Reconstr Surg 1975;55(6):682–6.

13. Chang BW, Luethke R, Berg WA, et al. Two- dimensional color Doppler imaging for precision preoperative mapping and size determination of TRAM flap perforators. Plast Reconstr Surg 1994;93(01):197–200.

14. Visconti G, Bianchi A, Hayashi A, et al. Designing An Anterolateral Thigh Flap Using Ultrasound. J Reconstr Microsurg 2022;38(3):206–16. https://doi.org/10.1055/s-0041-1740126.

15. Rozen WM, Phillips TJ, Stella DL, et al. Preoperative CT angiography for DIEP flaps: 'must-have' lessons for the radiolo- gist. J Plast Reconstr Aesthetic Surg 2009;62(12):e650–1.

16. Wade RG, Watford J, Wormald JCR, et al. Perforator mapping reduces the operative time of DIEP flap breast recon- struction: a systematic review and meta-analysis of preoperative ultrasound, computed tomography and magnetic resonance an- giography. J Plast Reconstr Aesthetic Surg 2018;71(04):468–77.

17. Rozen WM, Phillips TJ, Ashton MW, et al. Preoperative imaging for DIEA perforator flaps: a comparative study of computed tomographic angiography and Doppler ultra- sound. Plast Reconstr Surg 2008;121(01):9–16.

18. Aubry S, Pauchot J, Kastler A, et al. Preoperative imaging in the planning of deep inferior epigastric artery perforator flap surgery. Skeletal Radiol 2013;42(03):319–27.

19. Visconti G, Bianchi A, Di Leone A, et al. The Ultrasound Evolution of Lateral Thoracic Perforator Flaps Design and Harvest for Partial and Total Breast Reconstruction. Aesthetic Plast Surg 2024;48(5):894–904.

20. Salgarello M, Visconti G. Designing Lateral Thoracic Wall Perforator Flaps for Breast Reconstruction Using Ultrasound. J Reconstr Microsurg 2022;38(3):228–32.

21. Visconti G, Hayashi A. How to Find Perforator: Preoperative and Intraoperative. Part B: Color Duplex/Ultrasound. in Blondeel PN, et al. "Perforator Flaps: Technique & Clinical Applications". New York, USA: Thieme; 2023. p. 111–23.

22. Bianchi A, Visconti G, Hayashi A, et al. Ultra-High frequency ultrasound imaging of lymphatic channels correlates with their histological features: A step forward in lymphatic surgery. J Plast Reconstr Aesthetic Surg 2020;73(9):1622–9.

23. Visconti G, Salgarello M. Anteromedial thigh perforator-assisted closure of the anterolateral thigh free flap donor site. J Plast Reconstr Aesthetic Surg 2013;66(7):e189–92. Epub 2013 Mar 20. PMID: 23523166.

24. Visconti G, Yamamoto T, Hayashi N, et al. Ultrasound-Assisted Lymphaticovenular Anastomosis for the Treatment of Peripheral Lymphedema. Plast Reconstr Surg 2017;139(6):1380e–1e.

25. Visconti G, Hayashi A, Yoshimatsu H, et al. Ultra-high frequency ultrasound in planning capillary perforator flaps: Preliminary experience. J Plast Reconstr Aesthetic Surg 2018;71(8):1146–52.

26. Hayashi A, Giacalone G, Yamamoto T, et al. Ultra High-frequency Ultrasonographic Imaging with 70 MHz Scanner for Visualization of the Lymphatic Vessels. Plast Reconstr Surg Glob Open 2019;7(1):e2086.

27. Visconti G, Hayashi A, Tartaglione G, et al. Preoperative planning of lymphaticovenular anastomosis in patients with iodine allergy: A multicentric experience. J Plast Reconstr Aesthetic Surg 2020;73(4):783–808.

28. Bianchi A, Visconti G, Hayashi A, et al. Ultra-High frequency ultrasound imaging of lymphatic channels correlates with their histological features: A step

forward in lymphatic surgery. J Plast Reconstr Aesthetic Surg 2020;73(9):1622–9.

29. Hayashi A, Visconti G, Yamamoto T, et al. Intraoperative imaging of lymphatic vessel using ultra high-frequency ultrasound. J Plast Reconstr Aesthetic Surg 2018;71(5):778–80.

30. Visconti G, Bianchi A, Hayashi A, et al. Ultra-high frequency ultrasound preoperative planning of the rerouting method for lymphaticovenular anastomosis in incisions devoid of vein. Microsurgery 2020. https://doi.org/10.1002/micr.30600.

31. Visconti G, Salgarello M, Hayashi A. The Recipient Venule in Supermicrosurgical Lymphaticovenular Anastomosis: Flow Dynamic Classification and Correlation with Surgical Outcomes. J Reconstr Microsurg 2018;34(8):581–9.

32. Bianchi A, Salgarello M, Hayashi A, et al. Recipient Venule Selection and Anastomosis Configuration for Lymphaticovenular Anastomosis in Extremity Lymphedema: Algorithm Based on 1,000 Lymphaticovenular Anastomosis. J Reconstr Microsurg 2021. Epub ahead of print.

The Role of Computed Tomography Angiography in Perforator Flap Planning

Linda Chow, MD, FRCSC[a,1], Peter Dziegielewski, MD, FRCSC[b,2],
Harvey Chim, MD[c,*,3]

KEYWORDS

- Computed tomography angiography • Perforator mapping • Free flap • Head and neck
- Microsurgery

KEY POINTS

- Computed tomography angiography (CTA) is reliable, accurate, and precise in mapping and subsequently correlating perforators of medium to large size to the intraoperative domain.
- Preoperative CTA in perforator free-flap reconstruction enables a targeted harvesting of free flaps that can minimize donor site morbidity, with its ability to characterize the vascular anatomy and to identify vascular anomalies.
- CTA enables precise tailoring of the free-flap reconstruction to the defect, with applications in modifying the plane of dissection relative to perforator location—from the traditional subfascial plane, to the superficial fascia, to the subcutaneous plane—and in precise positioning of the virtual surgical planning cut guide relative to perforator location in bony reconstruction.
- Preoperative CTA in perforator flaps offers the potential to reduce operative time, with potential implications from a cost perspective.

BACKGROUND

Innovation in the world of microvascular free flaps is driven by the multifaceted aim of restoring as similar as possible what was "normal."[1] With functional considerations—particularly for head and neck defects, aesthetic considerations at the recipient site, and the essential consideration of donor site morbidity, perforator flaps have been explored extensively to achieve this overarching reconstructive goal.

A multitude of workhorse perforator flaps have been previously described, including, but not limited to, the deep inferior epigastric artery perforator (DIEP) flap, superficial inferior epigastric artery (SIEA) flap, superior gluteal artery perforator flap, anterolateral thigh (ALT) flap, anteromedial flap, and thoracodorsal artery perforator (TDAP) flap.

EVOLUTION OF COMPUTED TOMOGRAPHY ANGIOGRAPHY IN FLAP PLANNING

Owing to the inherent variability and complexity of the vascular anatomy of perforator flaps—not only between patients but also between the laterality of the soft tissues of a patient, the use of computed tomography angiography (CTA) was first applied by Masia and colleagues[2] in 2006 to

[a] Department of Otolaryngology–Head & Neck Surgery, University of Florida, Gainesville, FL, USA; [b] Advanced Head & Neck Oncologic Surgery, University of Florida, Gainesville, FL, USA; [c] Plastic Surgery and Neurosurgery, Division of Plastic and Reconstructive Surgery, Department of Surgery, University of Florida, PO Box 100138, Gainesville, FL 32610, USA
[1] Present address: 37 Harrison Road, Toronto, Ontario M2L 1V6, Canada.
[2] Present address: 4301 Southwest 96th Drive, Gainesville, FL 32608.
[3] Present addess: 4401 Southwest 105th Drive, Gainesville, FL 32608.
* Corresponding author. 1600 Southwest Archer Road, Gainesville, FL 32610.
E-mail address: harveychim@yahoo.com

Oral Maxillofacial Surg Clin N Am 36 (2024) 525–535
https://doi.org/10.1016/j.coms.2024.07.002
1042-3699/24/© 2024 Elsevier Inc. All rights reserved, including those for text and data mining, AI training, and similar technologies.

preoperatively evaluate the perforator anatomy of patients undergoing planned SIEA or DIEP breast reconstruction. CTA is a noninvasive imaging modality that is obtained over the approximate duration of 10 to 12 seconds over a single breath-hold in the supine patient,[2] while intravenous iodinated contrast is administered. Well-tolerated by the patient with the entire procedure duration less than 10 minutes, drawbacks to this modality include exposure to ionizing radiation and iodinated contrast medium,[3] cost,[2] and lack of information regarding flow characteristics.[4] After evaluating the perforator anatomy of both the DIEA and the SIEA systems of both hemi-abdomens in multiplanar and three-dimensional (3D) views, the study authors transposed this information to enable correlation with handheld Doppler ultrasound identification and intraoperative findings. Of their 66 cases of DIEP flaps with CTA, the study authors found no false positives or false negatives when comparing CTA with intraoperative findings. They further delineated a periumbilical region with the highest concentration of perforators, which continues to be used as an anatomic guide for identifying perforators of the DIEP system. Moreover, the findings of Masia and colleagues[2] of an average of 100 minutes of operative time saved per patient with the use of CTA compared with without the use of CTA has since been replicated by several studies to varying degrees.[5,6]

The work of Saint-Cyr and colleagues[7] subsequently helped elucidate the vascular anatomy and flow perfusion characteristics of the "perforasome," akin to Taylor and Palmer's angiosome concept.[8] With the aid of 3D and four-dimensional CTA and injection of dye directly into perforators and source vessels of 18 perforator flaps of the anterior trunk, posterior trunk, upper extremities, and lower extremities, Saint-Cyr and colleagues demonstrated 4 key principles: each perforator holds a unique vascular territory or "perforasome" that is multidirectional in flow and linked with adjacent perforasomes via direct and indirect linking vessels; the direction of the linking vessels can guide flap design and orientation; perforators of a single source artery preferentially fill first before perforators of another source artery; and vascularity of a perforator adjacent to an articulation is directed away from that same articulation.

Recognizing that an understanding of the vascular anatomy, and thus the vascular mapping, of a perforator flap is crucial to a flap's design and reconstructive utility, numerous imaging modalities have since been studied and compared. Comprehensive reviews by Smit and colleagues[9] and Ibelli and colleagues[3] on perforator mapping technologies both concluded the singular advantages of a

modality that can provide a 3D image of the perforator and vessel network anatomy, one chiefly provided by CTA. In addition, the detail with small-sized vessels offered by CTA remains unchallenged. Rozen and colleagues[10] conducted 2 studies to evaluate the accuracy of perforator mapping by CTA, one cadaveric and the other a prospective cohort study[11] of patients undergoing DIEP breast reconstruction. In the cadaveric study, CTA demonstrated an overall sensitivity of 96% and a positive predictive value (PPV) of 95% for mapping perforators; in addition, for perforators greater than 1 mm in diameter, the sensitivity was 100% and the PPV was 100%.[10] In the prospective cohort study, CTA identified 279 of a total of 280 major perforators, with a sensitivity of 99.6% and PPV of 99.6%.[11] Furthermore, when directly compared with its predecessor, the handheld Doppler ultrasound, and with magnetic resonance angiography (MRA), (1) CTA was more sensitive at identifying perforators and both the DIEP and the SIEA branching patterns[12]; and, (2) CTA was more sensitive in identifying the total number of perforators and the course of a perforator through soft tissue planes.[13]

COMPUTED TOMOGRAPHY ANGIOGRAPHY FOR SOFT TISSUE HEAD AND NECK RECONSTRUCTION

Beyond the extensive literature on CTA for DIEP breast reconstruction, there are comparatively fewer studies on the use of CTA for head and neck reconstruction. Perforator flaps for head and neck reconstruction for which CTA has been studied include the ALT flap,[14] medial sural artery perforator (MSAP) flap,[15] soleus perforator flap,[16] profunda artery perforator (PAP) flap,[17] TDAP,[18] superficial circumflex iliac artery perforator (SCIP),[19] and chimeric gracilis–PAP flap.[20]

Garvey and colleagues[14] were the first to prospectively compare CTA perforator mapping preoperatively compared with intraoperative perforator findings for the ALT flap for 16 patients with head and neck ablative defects, including laryngopharyngectomies, mandibulectomies, parotidectomies and temporal bone resections, and sinonasal disease resections. Using a line from the anterior superior iliac spine to the superior lateral patella, perforator distance was mapped until its entry point at the deep fascia, and subsequently compared with the intraoperative measurements. The mean difference of these 2 measurements was 3.5 mm. Overall sensitivity of CTA to identify a perforator was 74%, increasing to 92% for the proximal-most perforator, which is typically a larger perforator. In predicting the size of the perforators, accuracy of CTA was 68%, echoing similar findings of Rozen and colleagues[10–12] of a decrease in accuracy of CTA in identifying perforators of a smaller size, whereas overall accuracy of CTA in identifying a septocutaneous versus myocutaneous course was 78%. Notably, the study authors highlighted the impact of CTA in altering their surgical decision making in 38% of patients.[14] In these patients, CTA findings of the perforator origin (descending branch vs transverse branch of lateral circumflex femoral artery), origin of these source branches off the profunda femoris, or absence of perforators resulted in a modification to the harvesting of double-island flaps and use of the contralateral extremity. Overall, the study authors concluded that routine use of CTA for ALT flaps was not indicated but emphasized its utility whereby 2 skin paddles would be needed for more complex reconstruction.

This ability to plan a targeted harvesting of a perforator flap—particularly for complex defects requiring 2 skin paddles, is a key advantage echoed by a group investigating CTA for perforator mapping in TDAP reconstruction for the head and neck and the lower extremities.[18] The TDAP flap has historically relied on Doppler localization of perforators, with numerous influencing factors, including body habitus, body position, and the absence of fixed, anatomic landmarks. Mun and colleagues[18] compared CTA perforator mapping with Doppler flowmetry and intraoperative localization, demonstrating a 100% PPV in the premarked perforators, a statistically significant difference in operative time (77 minutes with preoperative CTA vs 101 minutes without CTA), and a significantly shorter surgical scar in patients with a TDAP flap with size less than 50 cm^2.

The reduced donor site morbidity has also been echoed by groups studying CTA in the soleus perforator flap for oral cavity carcinomas[16] and MSAP flap for T2-3 oral tongue carcinomas.[15] Perforator free flaps have variable perforator anatomy that may result in longer surgical incisions to ensure the ideal perforator is identified. Optimal oral cavity reconstruction is often achieved with the use of a pliable, thin skin paddle and long pedicle length with large-vessel diameter. Although the radial forearm free flap is a longstanding workhorse, its donor site morbidity is well-documented, giving rise to the exploration of perforator free flaps for medium-sized oral cavity ablative defects. For the reconstruction of oral tongue, buccal, and floor of mouth carcinomas, Wolff and colleagues[16] used CTA of the lower extremities to identify 12 of 20 patients with adequate perforator location, length, and caliber of the soleus perforator flap, a flap that often relies on intraoperative confirmation of the location of the perforator. The study authors

relied on CTA perforator mapping, supplemented by acoustic Doppler, to choose the laterality of the donor leg and the ideal perforator based on its position, length, and diameter. The study authors further described the selection of the soleus perforator flap based on the goal of achieving primary closure of the donor site and concluded that the need for microvascular anastomoses directly with perforator vessels mandates the use of preoperative perforator imaging.

ADVANCES IN PERFORATOR FLAPS WITH COMPUTED TOMOGRAPHY ANGIOGRAPHY

Beyond the value of CTA in its high sensitivity and accuracy for localizing large perforators, this imaging modality may help reconstructive surgeons create innovative approaches for the reconstruction of large, ablative defects with significant functional sequelae. In an article describing the radiologic characteristics of a dynamic, chimeric PAP-gracilis flap with a case report of its use after total glossectomy, Heredero and colleagues[20] used CTA to identify the first perforator of the adductor magnus joining with the main pedicle of the gracilis muscle. From there, the entry point of the perforator at the deep fascia was marked, and this location relative to the ischial tuberosity and gracilis was used to facilitate perforator identification intraoperatively. With the PAP flap component reconstituting neotongue bulk, supplemented by a portion of the gracilis muscle, and neurorrhaphy of the hypoglossal nerve to the obturator nerve, the study authors reported the patient tolerating an oral liquid diet on postoperative day 15, and electromyography studies demonstrating voluntary gracilis action 6 months after surgery.[20] Although these results are encouraging, this anatomic configuration to facilitate the chimeric flap was found in only 28% of imaged lower extremities. The study authors have nonetheless incorporated CTA and duplex ultrasound to their total glossectomy reconstructive algorithm to determine if this chimeric free flap is a viable option.

Since the first description of the ALT flap elevated in the superficial fascial plane[21] or the "thin" plane, various perforator flaps have been explored in this manner to both counteract the need for debulking procedures and tailor the donor flap to the defect. The PAP flap, harvested in traditional, subfascial fashion, was originally reported for breast reconstruction,[22] but was used subsequently by groups from Asian countries[23–25] for tongue reconstruction, a trend likely secondary to the larger bulk associated with thigh flaps associated with a higher body mass index (BMI) in non-Asian countries.[17] In applying the PAP flap for tongue reconstruction to a

Western population, Heredero and colleagues[17] described the preoperative use of CTA to design the flap based on the largest-diameter perforator and its location relative to the fixed landmark of the line between the ischial tuberosity and the superomedial patella border. In a cohort of 10 patients with T2-3 tongue carcinomas with a range of hemiglossectomy to subglossectomy and total glossectomy defects, the study authors customized the flap thickness by modifying the plane of dissection based on the ablative defect and the characteristics of the patient's thigh, while preserving the integrity of the identified perforator.

With sustained interest in the reconstructive surgeon's ability to tailor a flap's thickness to the defect, CTA has been used to further characterize the PAP flap perforator anatomy when harvesting in the thin and "superthin" planes, the latter of which is in the subcutaneous fat. With preoperative CTA perforator localization initially described in a series of 10 patients[25] and expanded on in a series of 80 patients,[26] 2 distinct PAP patterns were identified. In the "T" pattern, there is a superficial bifurcation of the perforator near the skin with the distal limbs traveling in a transverse fashion in the subdermal plane, whereas in the "Y" pattern, the perforator bifurcation is deeper near the deep fascia with its distal limbs traveling in an oblique fashion superficially.[26]

In the approach to identifying these 2 patterns,[26] the dominant perforator was first identified in the axial plane. The proximal-distal distance of the perforator was then measured at the midcoronal plane from groin crease to the exit site of the perforator from the deep fascia (**Fig. 1**A). Third, the "skin thickness" (defined as the distance from the fascia to the skin) (**Fig. 1**B) and the "thin thickness" (defined as the distance from the bifurcation point of the perforator to the skin) (**Fig. 1**C) were measured for the dominant perforator, allowing for calculation of a ratio of total skin thickness to "thin" thickness for

the dominant perforator. Preoperative CTA planning with a "Y" perforator pattern in a representative patient is shown in **Fig. 2**.

In this series[26] of 80 patients with 159 thighs evaluated for PAP flap reconstruction, the "T" perforator pattern (n = 97) was more common than the "Y" pattern (n = 62), with a greater skin thickness and "thin thickness" in female patients. The ratio thickness, however, was not associated with gender and only weakly associated with BMI, suggesting that the level at which the perforator bifurcates relative to the total skin thickness is constant.[26] When comparing the CTA measured "thin thickness" with its intraoperative value, there was a significant association for the "T" pattern, suggesting that the "T" perforator pattern predicts flap elevation at the superficial fascia or "thin" plane.

COMPUTED TOMOGRAPHY ANGIOGRAPHY FOR BONY HEAD AND NECK RECONSTRUCTION

In bony head and neck reconstruction, CTA has been used to precisely map the cutaneous perforators of osteocutaneous free flaps. In a prospective study of 40 patients undergoing fibula free flaps (FFF) for maxillary and mandibular defects, CTA was performed preoperatively, detecting 93 of 98 perforators, with no false positives.[27] Intraoperatively, all perforators on CTA were identified. Although CTA was less accurate in predicting perforator size, its accuracy in predicting the course of a perforator was 93%. Notably, the operative plan for 10 patients was modified based on the CTA findings, wherein the contralateral leg was chosen in 2 patients owing to hypoplastic posterior tibial arteries, and the proximal osteotomy was moved more cranial owing to the more proximal location of the tibioperoneal trunk.

CTA has been similarly applied for the deep circumflex iliac artery (DCIA) perforator flap in 5

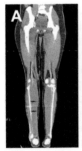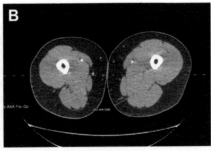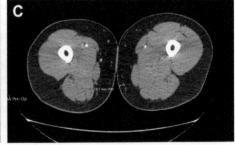

Fig. 1. Preoperative CTA planning of a representative patient with a dominant "T" pattern perforator in the left thigh. (*A*) Coronal view is used to measure proximal distal distance of the perforator. (*B*) Distance from deep fascia to the skin is measured. (*C*) Distance from bifurcation point of the perforator to the skin is measured. One limb of the "T" perforator can be seen in this image.

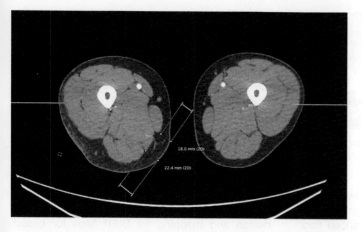

Fig. 2. Preoperative CTA planning of a representative patient with a dominant "Y" pattern perforator in the right thigh. Distance from deep fascia to the skin (*yellow*) and distance from bifurcation point of the perforator to the skin (*white*) are measured.

patients with head and neck defects.[28] In an effort to describe an alternative osteocutaneous free-flap option distinct from the workhouse FFF, the study authors found 7 of the 11 patients who underwent CTA demonstrated perforators with a diameter greater than 0.8 mm and an origin from the DCIA pedicle, consistent with previously published findings.[29] The investigators also reported the absence of long-term morbidities, including pain, paresthesias, necrosis, or fistula formation, although last follow-up with patients was reported to be at the 6-month postoperative period.

With advances in virtual surgical planning (VSP), CTA has been further demonstrated to accurately define perforator location and course relative to the planned location of the osteotomies using a VSP cut guide.[30–32] In a series[30] of 20 patients with planned FFF reconstruction for mandibular defects, CTA demonstrated aberrant vascular anatomy in 5 patients without clinical examination abnormalities. Two patients were found to have bilateral absence of the anterior tibial artery, precluding reconstruction with the FFF, and 3 patients required use of the contralateral leg owing to the origin of the dorsal arch from the peroneal artery. All CTA-identified perforators were identified intraoperatively, with a mean difference of perforator location at 1 mm (range, 0–2 mm). CTA localization enabled positioning of the VSP cut guide relative to the cutaneous perforators such that there was no modification of the planned osteotomies.

Ettinger and colleagues[32] expanded further on using CTA to optimally position the cut guide relative to the perforators in a prospective study of 60 patients undergoing FFF reconstruction. The investigators described marking the perforators at 2 locations: —(1) at the takeoff from the peroneal artery; and (2) at the crossing of the posterior border of the fibula.[33] From there, the locations of the osteotomies were planned such that the perforators were centralized on the bone segments. All

perforators incorporated into the reconstructive plan were identified intraoperatively, with no modifications to the virtual surgical plan made. CTA perforator localization demonstrated a 96% sensitivity, 98% specificity, 90% negative predictive value, and 99% PPV, with the technique most precise in the distal one-third of the leg with a median difference between CTA and intraoperative localization of 0.2 cm.

CASE STUDIES
Case 1: Thin Profunda Artery Perforator Flap

Following preoperative CTA planning with the addition of color Doppler ultrasound to localize the dominant PAP on the left thigh (see **Fig. 1**), a thin PAP flap was elevated (**Fig. 3**). Accurate localization of the dominant perforator allowed rapid and safe elevation of a PAP flap superficial to the Scarpa fascia, leaving most of the deep fat behind (see **Fig. 3**C).

Case 2: Chimeric Osteocutaneous Fibular Flap

Preoperative CTA imaging of the left leg showed an intramuscular soleus perforator from the peroneal artery perfusing the skin (**Fig. 4**A, B). An osteocutaneous free fibular flap was elevated with 2 skin paddles (**Fig. 4**C), proximal skin paddle based on the intramuscular soleus perforator seen in preoperative CTA and distal skin paddle based on a septocutaneous perforator. This allowed primary closure of the donor site in the left leg, while allowing coverage of a wider skin defect by rearranging the 2 skin paddles side by side.

Case 3: Anterolateral Thigh Flap

Correlating with acoustic handheld Doppler the day of surgery, the dominant myocutaneous perforator identified on CTA (**Fig. 5**A) was localized in a patient who required both an ALT free flap and

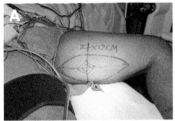
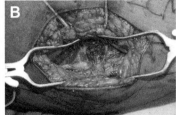
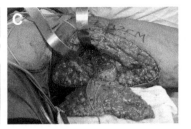

Fig. 3. Elevation of a thin PAP flap. Preoperative CTA planning was shown in **Fig. 1.** (*A*) Flap design. (*B*) Exposure of the dominant PAP. (*C*) Elevation of a PAP flap in the thin plane, leaving most of the deep fat behind in the donor site.

an FFF for reconstruction of the ablative external defect and inner mucosal and bony defect, respectively, from a very locally advanced floor-of-mouth squamous cell carcinoma invading the mandible and lower lip (**Fig. 5**B). CTA imaging facilitated rapid harvest of the flap in this complex ablative and reconstructive case.

Case 4: Osteocutaneous Fibula Free Flap for "Jaw-in-a-Day"

Preoperative CTA imaging (**Fig. 6**A, B) was used for VSP of the planned osteotomies and placement of dental implants in a patient requiring a segmental mandibulectomy. CTA further enabled the identification of a more proximally located perforator, which helped optimize the placement of the VSP cut guide relative to the perforator (**Fig. 6**C) and the positioning of the skin paddle relative to the dental prosthesis (**Fig. 6**D).

DISCUSSION

In the reconstructive surgeon's mission to replace like with like, CTA imaging has demonstrated broad clinical utility in a variety of perforator flaps. Extensively studied and validated, initially in the design and mapping for DIEP flaps for breast reconstruction, CTA has since been shown to be an effective tool for preoperative planning for head and neck reconstruction with the ALT flap, soleus perforator flap, TDAP, MSAP, SCIP, PAP, and FFF.

Specifically, CTA has been shown to be reliable, accurate, and precise in identifying and measuring perforators greater than 1.0 mm in diameter and in distinguishing the course of a perforator. Although multiple investigators[10,14] have reported on the decreased accuracy of CTA in identifying perforators less than 1.0 mm in diameter, it is important to recognize that this does not equate to the absence of perforators, which may subsequently be identified intraoperatively or identified with another modality like handheld Doppler. Moreover, the consistency of CTA in accurately depicting the course of a perforator has been suggested to be related to the encircling of perforators by subcutaneous fat.[14] Garvey and colleagues[14] found improved accuracy of CTA in identifying ALT flap

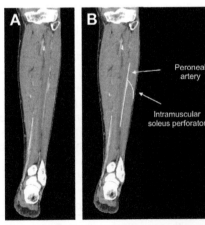
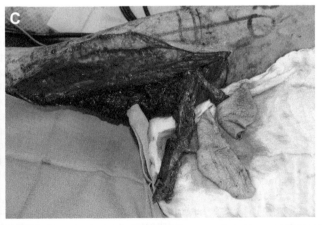

Fig. 4. Elevation of a double skin paddle chimeric fibular osteocutaneous flap. Intramuscular soleus perforator was visualized on preoperative coronal CTA images (*A, B*). (*C*) Two skin paddles elevated, proximal skin paddle perfused by intramuscular perforator seen preoperatively on CTA, distal skin paddle perfused by septocutaneous perforator.

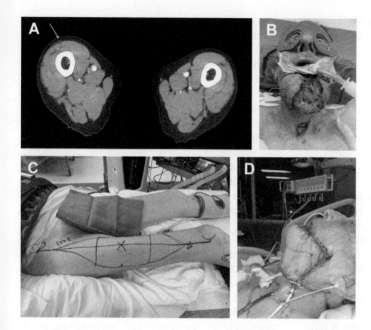

Fig. 5. Dominant myocutaneous perforator (*arrow*) of a right ALT flap, identified on preoperative CTA (*A*), in a patient who required both an ALT free flap and an FFF for reconstruction of the ablative external defect and inner mucosal and bony defect from a very locally advanced floor-of-mouth squamous cell carcinoma invading the mandible and lower lip (*B*). (*C*) Blue suture closest to the "x" is consistent with the identified perforator on CTA. (*D*) ALT skin paddle after inset, immediately postoperative.

perforators in patients with a higher BMI, suggesting this may account for the study's high sensitivity (92.3%) of CTA in identifying the proximal-most perforator. Studies comparing CTA to other imaging modalities, such as MRA[13] and handheld Doppler,[12] have further reinforced the superiority of CTA in delineating soft tissue planes and the course of perforators.

With its ability to map perforators accurately, CTA has enabled the targeted harvesting of free flaps based on one or more perforators. The ability to devise a precise, preoperative reconstructive plan for complex defects is a notable advantage of CTA, as demonstrated in its use for laryngopharyngectomies requiring double-paddle ALT flap reconstruction without the need for subsequent

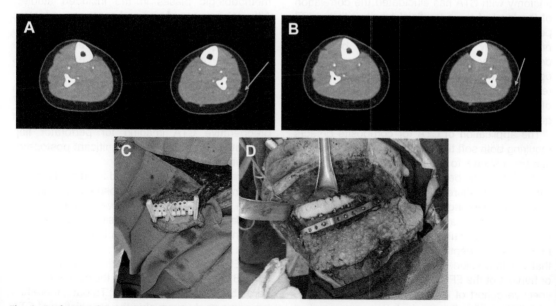

Fig. 6. Perforator (*arrows*) visualized on CTA of the left leg in an FFF for a segmental mandibulectomy (*A, B*). Its more proximal location identified on CTA helped plan the placement of the VSP cut guide (*C*) relative to the perforator. (*D*) The perforator, marked by the blue suture, supplying the skin paddle during inset of the free flap.

intraoperative modifications.[14] In turn, techniques commonly used to intraoperatively confirm the presence of a perforator, such as long surgical incisions to achieve wide exposure and harvesting of muscle, or the need to explore the contralateral extremity if a perforator is not identified, is often precluded. Multiple groups[15,16,18] have since demonstrated decreased donor site morbidity when comparing length of surgical scars or need for harvest of a skin graft between patients for whom preoperative CTA was and was not obtained.

Progression of technology and development of adjunctive tools, such as VSP, have resulted in opportunities for innovation with the use of CTA. In soft tissue reconstruction, CTA has helped push the boundaries of flap design and harvesting beyond the traditional subfascial plane. For a thigh-based flap influenced by body habitus and BMI, CTA has been used in the PAP flap to tailor flap thickness to that of the defect. In turn, this enables the use of this flap in patients with a high BMI, allowing patients to make use of the flap's advantage of a more concealed donor site incision and decreased likelihood of secondary flap debulking. With an increasing proportion of the global population with a BMI greater than 25 (ie, overweight) or BMI greater than 30 (ie, obese), with certain projections suggesting greater than 85% of adults in the United States by 2030,[33] such an expansion of the reconstructive surgeon's armamentarium is worthwhile.

Additional efforts to characterize the PAP flap anatomy with CTA has elucidated the correlation of the level of the superficial fascia with the "T" perforator pattern. With this knowledge gained preoperatively, flap elevation can be rapid, decreasing the duration of flap harvest and overall operative time while also enabling a more tailored reconstruction to that of the defect. The thickness of the PAP flap elevated can be tailored to the requirements of the defect.[34]

The application of CTA for composite defects requiring both soft tissue and bony reconstruction has been shown to be a practical and replicable tool[30–32] that can be incorporated into the existing infrastructure where VSP is used. In addition to accurately mapping the dominant perforators to the skin paddle relative to the planned osteotomy sites of the VSP cut guide in the osteocutaneous FFF, CTA can identify aberrant vascular anatomy that would preclude use of a particular extremity or harvest of the FFF itself. Interestingly, in a prospective cohort of 40 patients with preoperative CTA before FFF, the surgical plan was modified by the CTA findings in only 4 of the 11 patients who had had abnormal pulse examinations. Clinical examination did not consistently identify 2 patients with hypoplastic posterior tibial arteries, of whom one had normal, palpable pulses bilaterally, whereas the other patient did not.[27] The study authors did not recommend routinely obtaining a CTA before FFF, instead narrowing its indication for patients with abnormal pulse examinations or a history of arterial insufficiency.[27] In contrast, at the authors' institution, CTA of the lower extremities is obtained routinely for patients undergoing osteocutaneous free flaps for the purpose of VSP and confirming adequate three-vessel runoff in at least one lower extremity. In this vein, the impact of CTA on surgical decision making in perforator flaps for composite defects is overwhelmingly positive.

Beyond its immediate clinical utility, the impact of CTA on postoperative outcomes has been explored. Various groups[2,5,6,18] have reported a decrease in operative time when comparing patients for whom CTA was and was not used preoperatively in perforator flap reconstruction. A comprehensive systematic review and meta-analysis[35] of studies comparing operative time in DIEP for breast reconstruction in patients with and without preoperative imaging using CTA, MRA, or ultrasound found that mapping with CTA or MRA saved a mean of 54 minutes (3–105 minutes, 95% confidence interval). Risk of partial flap loss was 80% lower when CTA was used (relative risk, 0.2; 95% confidence interval, 0.04–0.6). However, the level of evidence was concluded to be low to very low with concerns of a high risk of methodologic biases in the included studies. Although sources of bias and confounding factors may not be adequately addressed in these studies, separate multi-institutional and database studies evaluating postoperative outcomes related to operative time have demonstrated associations of prolonged operative time with venous thromboembolism[36] and infection rates,[37] supporting further efforts to evaluate the impact of preoperative CTA imaging for perforator flap reconstruction on clinically significant postoperative outcomes.

Detractors of CTA have cited the modality's use of iodinated contrast and exposure to ionizing radiation as limiting factors. However, the potential sequelae, including hypersensitivity reactions to the contrast material and impact on renal function, is rare.[11] Exposure to ionizing radiation from CTA for DIEP flaps has been described to range from 5 to 5.6 mSv, which is less than the dose for a standard abdominal CT scan.[2,11,13] To date, there has been one study examining the association of CTA performed for perforator flaps, with cancer risk related to ionizing radiation exposure from the

CTA. In this 31-patient cohort[38] undergoing DIEP breast reconstruction, 19 patients underwent preoperative CTA. Mean radiation dose exposure from the CTA was 6.3 mSv (minimum, 2.1 mSv; maximum, 8.4 mSv), with mean prior cumulative radiation exposure of the entire cohort of 19.7 mSv. Using a radiation risk calculator available online from the American Society of Radiologic Technologists, the study authors found the risk of developing cancer from the CTA alone ranged from 1:1050 to 1:6030. It therefore remains important to recognize the contributions of a single CTA to a patient's cumulative ionizing radiation exposure and the implications thereof.

The financial costs of obtaining a CTA have been reported to be approximately $400[13] and $450[27] for that of the abdomen and lower extremities, respectively. A cost-utility analysis[38] of preoperative CTA for DIEP breast reconstruction compared with Doppler ultrasound found CTA to be more cost-effective than Doppler ultrasound, based on the postoperative outcomes of total flap loss, partial flap loss, and fat necrosis. Rates of these 3 complications reached statistical significance between the higher rates seen in Doppler ultrasound versus CTA, and sensitivity analysis evaluating the incremental cost-utility ratio based on operative time saved by CTA showed that CTA held a cost advantage when operative time was decreased by at least 21 minutes as compared with operative time with Doppler ultrasound. Furthermore, the investigators concluded that the clinical advantages held by CTA translated into CTA consistently representing the most cost-effective imaging modality, even in the absence of a reduction in operative time.[39] To the best of the authors' knowledge, this remains the only cost analysis performed for preoperative CTA in perforator flap reconstruction, and further studies are warranted to understand the cost implications in flaps other than the DIEP flap.

SUMMARY

Preoperative CTA for perforator free flaps is accurate, precise, and reliable in mapping perforator anatomy that can be used in the intraoperative domain. CTA holds important clinical value as a tool in surgical decision making and surgical innovation, enabling reconstructive surgeons to plan complex flap designs for extensive defects. Integration into existing infrastructures for VSP is feasible, and future efforts to characterize the association of preoperative CTA with postoperative outcomes and cost-analyses for perforator flaps, beyond the DIEP flap, are warranted.

CLINICS CARE POINTS

- Computed tomography angiography imaging is a validated tool in defining the vascular anatomy of perforator free flaps.
- The application of preoperative computed tomography angiography to the reconstruction of complex defects, be it soft tissue, bony, or composite, holds tremendous value in centering a surgical reconstructive plan and aiding surgical decision making.
- Advances in technology combined with computed tomography angiography have enabled innovation in perforator free flaps in the form of virtual surgical planning and harvesting of perforator flaps in the superficial fascial and subcutaneous planes.
- Areas of further exploration include cost-analyses and characterizing the association of preoperative computed tomography angiography with postoperative outcomes in perforator free flaps.

DISCLOSURES

The authors have nothing to disclose.

REFERENCES

1. Millard DR Jr. Tissue losses should be replaced in kind. In: Millard DR, editor. Principlization of plastic surgery. Boston: Little, Brown; 1986. p. 191–228.
2. Masia J, Clavero JA, Larrañaga JR, et al. Multidetector-row computed tomography in the planning of abdominal perforator flaps. J Plast Reconstr Aesthetic Surg 2006;59(6):594–9.
3. Ibelli TJ, Chennareddy S, Mandelbaum M, et al. Vascular mapping for abdominal-based breast reconstruction: a comprehensive review of current and upcoming imaging modalities. Eplasty 2023; 23:e44. PMID: 37664815; PMCID: PMC10472443.
4. Thiessen FEF, Vermeersch N, Tondu T, et al. Dynamic Infrared Thermography (DIRT) in DIEP flap breast reconstruction: A clinical study with a standardized measurement setup. Eur J Obstet Gynecol Reprod Biol 2020;252:166–73.
5. Smit JM, Dimopoulou A, Liss AG, et al. Preoperative CT angiography reduces surgery time in perforator flap reconstruction. J Plast Reconstr Aesthetic Surg 2009;62(9):1112–7.
6. Haddock NT, Dumestre DO, Teotia SS. Efficiency in DIEP flap breast reconstruction: the real benefit of computed tomographic angiography imaging. Plast Reconstr Surg 2020;146(4):719–23.

7. Saint-Cyr M, Wong C, Schaverien M, et al. The perforasome theory: vascular anatomy and clinical implications. Plast Reconstr Surg 2009;124(5):1529–44.

8. Taylor GI, Palmer JH. The vascular territories (angiosomes) of the body: experimental study and clinical applications. Br J Plast Surg 1987;40(2):113–41.

9. Smit JM, Klein S, Werker PM. An overview of methods for vascular mapping in the planning of free flaps. J Plast Reconstr Aesthetic Surg 2010; 63(9):e674–82.

10. Rozen WM, Ashton MW, Stella DL, et al. The accuracy of computed tomographic angiography for mapping the perforators of the DIEA: a cadaveric study. Plast Reconstr Surg 2008;122(2):363–9.

11. Rozen WM, Ashton MW, Stella DL, et al. The accuracy of computed tomographic angiography for mapping the perforators of the deep inferior epigastric artery: a blinded, prospective cohort study. Plast Reconstr Surg 2008;122(4):1003–9.

12. Rozen WM, Phillips TJ, Ashton MW, et al. Preoperative imaging for DIEA perforator flaps: a comparative study of computed tomographic angiography and Doppler ultrasound. Plast Reconstr Surg 2008; 121(1):9–16.

13. Rozen WM, Stella DL, Bowden J, et al. Advances in the pre-operative planning of deep inferior epigastric artery perforator flaps: magnetic resonance angiography. Microsurgery 2009;29(2):119–23.

14. Garvey PB, Selber JC, Madewell JE, et al. A prospective study of preoperative computed tomographic angiography for head and neck reconstruction with anterolateral thigh flaps. Plast Reconstr Surg 2011;127(4):1505–14.

15. He Y, Jin SF, Zhang ZY, et al. A prospective study of medial sural artery perforator flap with computed tomographic angiography-aided design in tongue reconstruction. J Oral Maxillofac Surg 2014;72(11):2351–65.

16. Wolff KD, Bauer F, Dobritz M, et al. Further experience with the free soleus perforator flaps using CT-angiography as a planning tool - a preliminary study. J Cranio-Maxillo-Fac Surg 2012;40(8):e253–7.

17. Heredero S, Sanjuan A, Falguera MI, et al. The thin profunda femoral artery perforator flap for tongue reconstruction. Microsurgery 2020;40(2):117–24.

18. Mun GH, Kim HJ, Cha MK, et al. Impact of perforator mapping using multidetector-row computed tomographic angiography on free thoracodorsal artery perforator flap transfer. Plast Reconstr Surg 2008; 122(4):1079–88.

19. He Y, Tian Z, Ma C, et al. Superficial circumflex iliac artery perforator flap: identification of the perforator by computed tomography angiography and reconstruction of a complex lower lip defect. Int J Oral Maxillofac Surg 2015;44(4):419–23.

20. Heredero S, Falguera-Uceda MI, Sanjuan-Sanjuan A, et al. Chimeric profunda artery perforator - gracilis flap: A computed tomographic angiography study and case report. Microsurgery 2021;41(3):250–7.

21. Hong JP, Chung IW. The superficial fascia as a new plane of elevation for anterolateral thigh flaps. Ann Plast Surg 2013;70(2):192–5.

22. Allen RJ, Haddock NT, Ahn CY, et al. Breast reconstruction with the profunda artery perforator flap. Plast Reconstr Surg 2012;129(1):16e–23e.

23. Scaglioni MF, Kuo YR, Yang JC, et al. The posteromedial thigh flap for head and neck reconstruction: anatomical basis, surgical technique, and clinical applications. Plast Reconstr Surg 2015;136(2):363–75.

24. Wu JC, Huang JJ, Tsao CK, et al. Comparison of posteromedial thigh profunda artery perforator flap and anterolateral thigh perforator flap for head and neck reconstruction. Plast Reconstr Surg 2016; 137(1):257–66.

25. Chim H. The superthin profunda artery perforator flap for extremity reconstruction: clinical implications. Plast Reconstr Surg 2022;150(4):915–8.

26. Chim H. Suprafascial radiological characteristics of the superthin profunda artery perforator flap. J Plast Reconstr Aesthetic Surg 2022;75(7):2064–9.

27. Garvey PB, Chang EI, Selber JC, et al. A prospective study of preoperative computed tomographic angiographic mapping of free fibula osteocutaneous flaps for head and neck reconstruction. Plast Reconstr Surg 2012;130(4):541e–9e.

28. Ting JW, Rozen WM, Chubb D, et al. Improving the utility and reliability of the deep circumflex iliac artery perforator flap: the use of preoperative planning with CT angiography. Microsurgery 2011; 31(8):603–9.

29. Ting JW, Rozen WM, Grinsell D, et al. The in vivo anatomy of the deep circumflex iliac artery perforators: defining the role for the DCIA perforator flap. Microsurgery 2009;29(4):326–9.

30. Battaglia S, Maiolo V, Savastio G, et al. Osteomyocutaneous fibular flap harvesting: Computer-assisted planning of perforator vessels using Computed Tomographic Angiography scan and cutting guide. J Cranio-Maxillo-Fac Surg 2017;45(10):1681–6.

31. Ettinger KS, Alexander AE, Arce K. Computed tomographic angiography perforator localization for virtual surgical planning of osteocutaneous fibular free flaps in head and neck reconstruction. J Oral Maxillofac Surg 2018;76(10):2220–30.

32. Ettinger KS, Morris JM, Alexander AE, et al. Accuracy and precision of the computed tomographic angiography perforator localization technique for virtual surgical planning of composite osteocutaneous fibular free flaps in head and neck reconstruction. J Oral Maxillofac Surg 2022;80(8):1434–44.

33. Wang Y, Beydoun MA, Liang L, et al. Will all Americans become overweight or obese? Estimating the progression and cost of the US obesity epidemic. Obesity 2008;16(10):2323–30.

34. Chim H. Perforator mapping and clinical experience with the superthin profunda artery perforator flap for reconstruction in the upper and lower extremities. J Plast Reconstr Aesthetic Surg 2023;81:60–7.

35. Wade RG, Watford J, Wormald JCR, et al. Perforator mapping reduces the operative time of DIEP flap breast reconstruction: a systematic review and meta-analysis of preoperative ultrasound, computed tomography and magnetic resonance angiography. J Plast Reconstr Aesthetic Surg 2018;71(4):468–77.

36. Mlodinow AS, Khavanin N, Ver Halen JP, et al. Increased anaesthesia duration increases venous thromboembolism risk in plastic surgery: A 6-year analysis of over 19,000 cases using the NSQIP dataset. J Plast Surg Hand Surg 2015;49(4):191–7.

37. Daley BJ, Cecil W, Clarke PC, et al. How slow is too slow? Correlation of operative time to complications: an analysis from the Tennessee Surgical Quality Collaborative. J Am Coll Surg 2015;220(4):550–8.

38. Eylert G, Deutinger M, Stemberger A, et al. Evaluation of the perforator CT-angiography with a cancer risk assessment in DIEP flap breast reconstruction. J Plast Reconstr Aesthetic Surg 2015;68(4):e80–2.

39. Offodile AC 2nd, Chatterjee A, Vallejo S, et al. A cost-utility analysis of the use of preoperative computed tomographic angiography in abdomen-based perforator flap breast reconstruction. Plast Reconstr Surg 2015;135(4):662e–9e. Erratum in: Plast Reconstr Surg. 2015 Sep;136(3):626.

Thinned Perforator Flaps in Head and Neck Reconstruction

Jeremy Mingfa Sun, MBBS, MRCS, MMed, FAMS[a],
Takumi Yamamoto, MD, PhD[b],*

KEYWORDS

• Thinned • Superthin • Ultrathin • Perforator flaps • Pure skin perforator

KEY POINTS

• Thinned perforator flaps are now considered mainstream options in head and neck reconstruction.
• Although secondary thinning of perforator flaps is safest, primary thinning achieved through suprafascial elevation is gaining popularity as surgeons understand the vascular anatomy better.
• Pen Doppler, Doppler ultrasound, and Computed Tomographic angiography are useful adjuncts that help in preoperative perforator localization, making thinned flap elevation safer and more expedient.
• Thinned flaps can be used for a wide variety of indications in head and neck reconstruction.

EVOLUTION OF PERFORATOR FLAPS

Flap reconstruction has enjoyed a long, illustrious history, beginning with Sushruta utilizing the forehead flap for nasal reconstruction to Sir Harold Gilles' tubed pedicled flaps during World War 1 and 2. The history of perforator flaps is comparatively infantile. Pioneers such as Manchot[1] and Salmon[2] performed cadaveric studies that turned the spotlight on larger cutaneous arteries that emerged between fissures of the muscle and deep fascia. In 1989, Koshima and Soeda used the term "perforator flap" for the first time in a clinical setting.[3] They utilized a periumbilical perforator to harvest a flap for groin and tongue reconstruction. This served as the basis for Robert Allen's work on the deep inferior epigastric artery perforator flap that is now popular for breast reconstruction.[4] The sudden interest in perforator flaps led to much confusion in the terminology.

The "Gent" consensus was thus drawn up to standardize the terminology used in this subspecialized field of flap reconstruction.[5]

With advancing technology in imaging, surgical instruments, optics, and sutures, perforator flap harvest became less demanding yet more precise on a microvascular level. Flap survival has progressed to be consistently high. This has led to the quest for thinner and more bespoke flaps with various tissue components to accomplish the "perfect" reconstruction. The anterolateral thigh (ALT) flap and the superficial circumflex iliac artery perforator (SCIP) flap are now 2 of the most commonly performed flaps globally, owing to their consistent vascular anatomy and ease of flap harvest. The popularity of suprafascial perforator flaps has also risen exponentially since the article by Goh and Hong in 2015.[6] Consequently, an increasing number of surgeons are now exploring the harvest of flaps located superficial to the

[a] Plastic, Reconstructive and Aesthetic Surgery Service, Department of Surgery, Changi General Hospital, 2 Simei Street 3, Singapore 529889, Singapore; [b] Department of Plastic and Reconstructive Surgery, Center Hospital of National Center for Global Health and Medicine, 1-21-1 Toyama, Shinjuku-ku, Tokyo 162-8655, Japan
* Corresponding author.
E-mail address: tyamamoto-tky@umin.ac.jp

Oral Maxillofacial Surg Clin N Am 36 (2024) 537–544
https://doi.org/10.1016/j.coms.2024.07.013
1042-3699/24/© 2024 Elsevier Inc. All rights reserved, including those for text and data mining, AI training, and similar technologies.

superficial fascia, including those within the superficial fat or even the subdermal planes, commonly referred to as "pure skin perforator" flaps.[7,8]

CLASSIFICATION AND DEFINITIONS OF THINNED FLAPS

Much like the ongoing debates surrounding the definition of a perforator, the terminology employed for describing the planes of elevation needs to be more consistent. Sakarya and colleagues observed this disparity in the Asian and Western literature.[9] The historical origins of the term "superthin flap" can be traced back to Chinese surgeons Wang and colleagues and Sun and colleagues.[10,11] Subsequently, this terminology gained prominence through the work of Drs Hyakusoku and Narushima.[7,12] Flaps were classified based on their thickness as follows:

1. Myocutaneous flap: The flap is harvested with all layers of the skin, subcutaneous tissue, muscle fascia, and muscle.
2. Fasciocutaneous flap: The flap is harvested with all layers of the skin, subcutaneous tissue, and the deep muscle fascia. No muscle is harvested with the flap.
3. Perforator flap: The flap is harvested without including the deep muscle fascia and muscle.
4. Thin flap: The flap is elevated through the superficial (Scarpa's) fascia. Deep fat is not included in the flap.
5. Superthin flap: The flap is elevated through the superficial fat, leaving the subdermal vascular plexus intact (**Fig. 1**).
6. Pure skin perforator flap: The flap is harvested without any superficial fat and relies on the

pure skin perforator through its deep dermal plexus to provide sufficient perfusion.

Kwon and Hong from Asian Medical Center attempted to standardize the definitions used for the elevation planes.[13] The 5 types of perforator flaps based on their plane of elevation are as follows:

1. Subfascial flap: The flap is harvested with the deep muscle fascia attached. The plane of elevation is deep to the deep muscle fascia.
2. Suprafascial flap: The flap is harvested with the entire thickness of the subcutaneous tissue layer but without the deep muscle fascia attached. The plane of elevation is superficial to the deep muscle fascia.
3. Superthin flap: The flap is harvested with only the superficial fat attached. The elevation plane is through the loose superficial (Scarpa's) fascia.
4. Ultrathin flap: The flap is harvested with a split-thickness portion of the superficial fat. The elevation plane is through the superficial fat and the "pseudo-fascia." This pseudo-fascia dissection requires dissecting between lobules of superficial fat where loose fascia-like tissue exists.
5. Pure skin perforator flap: The flap is harvested without any superficial fat and relies on the pure skin perforator through its deep dermal plexus to provide sufficient perfusion. The plane of elevation is subdermal.

Standardization of the terminology is still required to ensure future clarity for surgeons.

Vascularity of the flap is often the most significant concern when elevating thinned flaps. Saint-Cyr demonstrated that direct and indirect linking vessels that link adjacent perforasomes are located within the subcutaneous tissue.[14] Through their studies, the Asian Medical Center group believes that many of these direct and indirect linking vessels exist in the superficial fat, which explains the reliability of superthin flaps.

PRE-OPERATIVE PLANNING FOR THINNED PERFORATOR FLAPS

The evolution of pre-operative planning and perforator mapping has closely followed the increasing complexities of flap reconstruction. As reconstructive surgeons seek thinner flaps with diverse tissue components, there is a growing demand for modalities offering precision, speed, and scalability.

The highly portable and cost-effective handheld pen Doppler maintains prominence among the tools commonly employed for perforator mapping

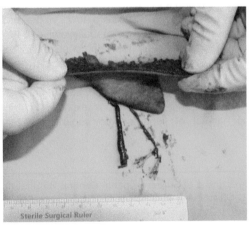

Fig. 1. The figure shows the elevation of a superficial circumflex iliac artery perforator (SCIP) flap through the superficial fat. The super-thin flap has only 1 globular layer of fat.

and flap design. While effective, it falls short in distinguishing a perforator from its larger source vessel and identifying dominant perforators, thus resulting in a relatively high rate of false positives.[15] Nevertheless, the pen Doppler is suitable for basic perforator localization in subfascial and suprafascial flaps.[16]

In contrast, Computed Tomography Angiography (CTA) and Doppler Ultrasound (DUS) stand out as the current advanced modalities for precise perforator localization and recipient vessel assessment. CTA excels in accurately pinpointing the location of all significant perforators and their surrounding anatomy. It allows observation of a perforator's branching pattern and intramuscular route through serial images, with the added benefit of quick performance and minimal interobserver variability.[17] However, it comes with the drawbacks of cost and the requirement for ionizing radiation. DUS, especially with higher frequency models (15Mhz and above), has the capability to map perforator locations and their courses to the skin without exposing patients to ionizing radiation (**Fig. 2**). This is particularly critical for surgeons raising superthin, ultrathin, and pure skin perforator (PSP) flaps, as precise knowledge of the point where the perforator traverses (**Fig. 3**) the plane of elevation is essential to avoid pedicle injury.[8] DUS in color mode offers real-time visualization, allowing surgeons to mark this crucial point on the patient. Notably, proficient utilization of DUS for this purpose necessitates time, training, and practice.

It is advisable for reconstructive surgeons working with thinned flaps to consider these tools during pre-operative planning.

THE TECHNIQUE OF FLAP THINNING
Primary Flap Thinning

Suprafascial flap harvest has gained popularity as it is quick and practical. Thinned flaps can be raised at the different planes as described earlier, but surgeons need to keep in mind the limitations and potential pitfalls of such harvest as well.

1. Inexperienced surgeons may inadvertently damage perforators during dissection as the caliber of these perforators tends to be much smaller than at the subfascial level. This is especially so for subdermal dissection of PSP flaps, as this requires experience to discern which are the dominant vessels to the skin.
2. As the flap is thinned increasingly, it relies more on indirect linking vessels than direct linking vessels. This moderated perfusion requires a surgeon to design smaller flaps to reduce the

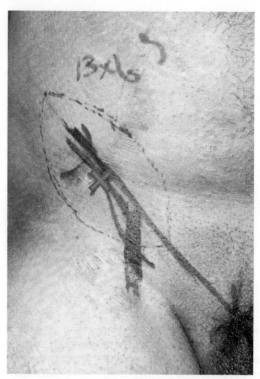

Fig. 2. Markings of the superficial branch of the superficial circumflex iliac artery perforator flap. The point at which the perforator (*red line*) pierces the superficial (Scarpa's) fascia is marked "X" and was located using ultrasonography. This correlated well intraoperatively with the position of the perforator. In addition, the superficial circumflex iliac vein was also traced and mapped on the skin.

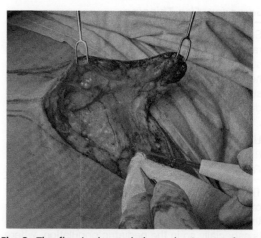

Fig. 3. The flap is elevated above the Scarpa's fascia leaving only a thin layer of superficial fat attached to the dermis. Knowing where the perforator pierces the Scarpa's fascia allows for safe and expedient dissection.

incidence of partial necrosis. However, there is little consensus on the appropriate size for each type of thinned flap. Indocyanine green angiography is a useful intra-operative adjunct for determining the appropriate size of the flap.[18–20]

3. Accurate preoperative mapping of the perforator, as it travels in the superficial fat, allows the surgeon to site the perforator at the center of the skin paddle. An eccentrically sited perforator will affect the flap's perfusion.[21]

4. It is technically more demanding to harvest thinned flaps with multiple perforators.

5. In a systematic review of flap thinning techniques,[22] suprafascial flap elevation of anterolateral thigh flaps had significantly higher vascular complications (10.4%), such as partial necrosis, marginal necrosis, and total flap loss, compared to subfascial elevation and subsequent defatting (3.1%).

Microdissection involves skeletonizing the perforator supplying the flap using a microscope.[23] The fat is carefully removed around the pedicle, preserving as many perforator branches as possible. This is done using meticulous microsurgical techniques and can be time-consuming. The risk of accidental damage to the smaller branches is also present.

Defatting is considered a reliable method of primary flap thinning. This involves elevating the flap at the subfascial plane, followed by lipectomy via sharp excision or diathermy. This technique preserves the deep fascia and the entire thickness of subcutaneous tissue with a 3.5 cm radius around the perforator.[24]

Secondary Flap Thinning

Secondary flap thinning is accomplished separately from the index flap reconstruction.[25] The surgeon waits a few months to allow the flap to heal into the recipient site, augmenting its blood supply. Liposuction and direct excision are used during secondary thinning (**Fig. 4**).

UTILITY IN HEAD AND NECK RECONSTRUCTION
Facial and Scalp Reconstruction

The facial and scalp skin is thin and pliable, and often, conventional perforator flaps cannot match the soft tissue thickness of the recipient site. This is especially so in the pediatric population, where the usual donor sites like the anterolateral thigh have significant adiposity, thus requiring thinned flaps. The scalp, forehead, nasal, and perioral regions are challenging as defects can be large or

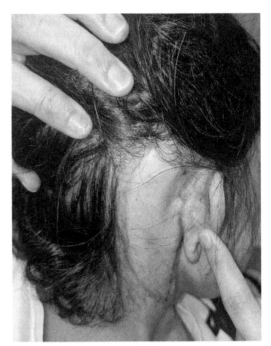

Fig. 4. Secondary thinning using liposuction of an anterolateral thigh flap postoperative day 10. The caudal portion of the flap required most of the debulking as it carried the perforator and the vascular pedicle.

require very thin soft tissue coverage. While the radial forearm flap is often used for perioral reconstruction, nasal reconstruction, and reconstruction of minor facial defects, the size of the radial forearm flap is often the limiting factor.[26]

The thinned ALT flap can resurface the whole forehead, while the superthin SCIP has been used to reconstruct the lips, malar skin, and eyelids.[27] For nasal reconstruction, a few authors have attempted to use thinned ALT, SCIP, and even superficial inferior epigastric artery perforator flaps.[28,29] However, in total nasal reconstruction, Burget and Walton described their technique of using free radial forearm flaps for inner lining reconstruction, cartilage grafts for structural integrity, and extended forehead flaps for superficial resurfacing.[30] Their elegant technique demonstrated superior esthetic outcomes and high patient satisfaction.

Tongue Reconstruction

The main goals of tongue reconstruction are to preserve speech and swallowing function. If the floor of the mouth is resected as well, then the flap separates the oral cavity from the neck and obliterates any dead space. While the flap used to reconstruct the tongue tip needs to be thin and pliable, significant bulk is required if the base of the tongue is to be reconstructed. The radial forearm flap is regarded as the workhorse for tongue reconstruction, especially for hemiglossectomies and lesser.[31] Several authors described the suprafascial radial forearm flap, which preserves the deep muscle fascia, leading to improved skin graft take and reduced donor site morbidity.[32,33] However, the scars are still unesthetic and in a highly visible area. Scar contractures still occur, albeit less than traditional radial forearm flaps.

Surgeons have adapted by using thinned flaps for tongue reconstruction to overcome these drawbacks of the radial forearm flap. The suprafascial and superthin ALT is often reported in the literature as the viable alternative to the suprafascial radial forearm flap. The ability to provide bulk in areas like the base of the tongue and the floor of the mouth, while also thinning the flap distilling to give the tongue tip mobility can be seen as an advantage. The donor site is also known to have significantly less morbidity than the radial forearm flap.[34] Despite this, there is yet to be a clear winner when comparing functional outcomes.[31]

The SCIP flap has also been increasingly described for tongue reconstruction.[27,35] The SCIP flap is a very versatile flap where multiple chimeric components such as skin, nerve, bone, and fascia can be raised. Furthermore, the thickness can be customized according to the defect. Like previous flap comparative studies, the SCIP flap does not have any clear advantage over the ALT or the Radial forearm flap.[36] Other flaps, such as the thinned peroneal artery perforator flap, have also been described for tongue reconstruction.[37]

Intraoral Resurfacing

Other than tongue reconstruction, thinned flaps can resurface the buccal mucosa, palate,[38] and, not so commonly, the nasopharynx. As nasopharyngeal carcinomas are usually treated with primary radiotherapy, flap reconstruction is uncommon.

However, when recurrences occur, a thinned flap may sometimes be used to resurface the area and cover the exposed carotid vessels.[39]

Maxillary Reconstruction

Maxillary reconstruction often requires soft tissue bulk to obliterate dead space. That is why thinned flaps are not usually considered for this indication. However, some surgeons utilize chimeric flaps where some skin paddles are thinned to match the surrounding tissue, like the facial skin or the palate. Combined superficial and deep branch chimeric SCIP flaps exemplify this indication. Yamamoto and colleagues used the bulkier skin paddle to obliterate the dead space of the maxillary sinus while utilizing the thinned skin paddle for palate lining.[40]

External Auditory Canal Reconstruction

Resurfacing the external auditory canal represents the pinnacle of thinned flaps. As the skin and soft tissue lining the external auditory canal are tubed and extremely thin, a pliable flap with almost no subcutaneous tissue is required to prevent the passageway from being occluded.

Narushima and colleagues described a pure skin perforator SCIP flap for reconstructing the external auditory canal to treat microtia and congenital aural atresia.[41,42] The pure skin perforator SCIP flap was thinned through microdissection, which was tedious and time-consuming. Yamamoto and colleagues demonstrated that a subdermal dissection technique can be used to raise pure skin perforator flaps safely and more expediently.[8]

Occasionally, patients require excision and obliteration of the entire external auditory canal. **Fig. 5** illustrates this case in a middle-aged lady with squamous cell carcinoma of the external auditory canal. Wide excision was done together with a limited temporal bone excision. Reconstruction was done with an SCIP flap elevated within the layer of the deep fat to preserve some flap bulk for dead space obliteration.

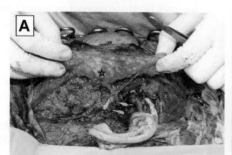 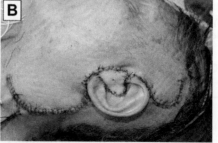

Fig. 5. (A) Shows an SCIP flap where the deep fat (*star*) was preserved in the central portion of the flap to obliterate dead space. (B) Shows a pleasing contour post-operatively.

	Anterolateral Thigh Flap	Superficial Circumflex Iliac Artery Perforator Flap	Radial Forearm Flap
Table 1 **A quick reference guide comparing the characteristics of popular thinned perforator flaps**			
Pedicle length	Long (can be longer than 10 cm)	Short to moderate (approximately 6 cm)	Long (can be longer than 10 cm)
Chimeric flap	Muscle, nerve, fascia	Muscle, nerve, fascia, bone,	Bone, nerve
Artery caliber	Large	Small	Large
Customizable thickness	Highly customizable	Highly customizable	Low customizability
Pure skin perforator flap	Not described	Described	Not described
Size of skin paddle	Large	Moderate	Small
Learning curve	Low	High	Low
Risk of donor site contracture	Low	Low	Moderate
Donor site scar and appearance	Good, concealed	Excellent, well concealed scar	Visible forearm scarring

SUMMARY

In conclusion, the evolution of perforator flaps in head and neck reconstruction has brought about significant advancements in surgical techniques and outcomes. The journey from the early pioneering studies by Manchot and Salmon to the establishment of standardized nomenclature through the "Gent" consensus has paved the way for developing thinner and more specialized perforator flaps.

Pre-operative planning, aided by modalities such as Computed Tomography Angiography (CTA) and Doppler Ultrasound (DUS), has become increasingly accurate and efficient. These tools help surgeons pinpoint perforator locations and design flaps with precision, which is crucial when working with thinned flaps.

As technology advances and surgical techniques evolve, the future of head and neck reconstruction holds even greater promise for achieving optimal results with thinned perforator flaps. The authors have provided **Table 1** as a quick reference guide to the features of commonly used thinned flaps in head and neck reconstruction.

CLINICS CARE POINTS

- The high-frequency Doppler ultrasound provides real-time localization of the perforator emergence point through the superficial fascia. This makes flap elevation safer and faster.

- Flap thinning reduces the vascularity of the flap making the edges prone to ischemia. Indocyanine green angiography is a useful intra-operative adjunct to reduce the probability of this happening after flap inset.

- When the flap's vascularity is doubtful, secondary thinning can be performed later to maximize the flap surface area and reduce the risk of partial flap necrosis.

- The surgeon's ability to customize the thickness of the flap to suit the reconstruction allows him or her to enhance both functional and esthetic outcomes.

DISCLOSURES

Authors have nothing to disclose.

REFERENCES

1. Manchot C. The cutaneous arteries of the human body. NY: Springer-Verlag; 1983. p. 136–7.
2. Cormack GC, Lamberty BG. The arterial anatomy of skin flaps. Edinburgh (United Kingdom): Churchill Livingstone; 1994.
3. Koshima I, Soeda S. Inferior epigastric artery skin flaps without rectus abdominis muscle. Br J Plast Surg 1989;42(6):645–8.
4. Allen RJ, Treece P. Deep inferior epigastric perforator flap for breast reconstruction. Ann Plast Surg 1994;32(1):32–8.
5. Blondeel PN, Van Landuyt KH, Monstrey SJ, et al. The "Gent" consensus on perforator flap terminology:

preliminary definitions. Plast Reconstr Surg 2003; 112(5):1378–83 [quiz 1383, 1516; discussion 1384-7].

6. Goh TLH, Park SW, Cho JY, et al. The search for the ideal thin skin flap: superficial circumflex iliac artery perforator flap–a review of 210 cases. Plast Reconstr Surg 2015;135(2):592–601.

7. Narushima M, Yamasoba T, Iida T, et al. Pure skin perforator flaps: the anatomical vascularity of the superthin flap. Plast Reconstr Surg 2018;142(03): 351e–60e.

8. Yamamoto T, Yamamoto N, Fuse Y, et al. Subdermal Dissection for Elevation of Pure Skin Perforator Flaps and Superthin Flaps: The Dermis as a Landmark for the Most Superficial Dissection Plane. Plast Reconstr Surg 2021;147(3):470–8.

9. Sakarya AH, Do N. Nomenclature of Thin and Super-Thin Flaps-Comment on: Outcomes of Subfascial, Suprafascial, and Super-Thin Anterolateral Thigh Flaps: Tailoring Thickness without Added Morbidity. J Reconstr Microsurg 2018;34(3):e3–4.

10. Wang Y-J, Zhang F-Q, Yang C-W, et al. Clinical application of early division of the pedicle of the super-thin flap with a subdermal vascular network. Practical Journal of Aesthetic and Plastic Surgery (Chinese) 1990;1:23–4.

11. Sun Y-H, Wang C-Y, Li C, et al. A study of the blood circulation of the "super-thin" skin flap with a preserved subdermal vascular network and its clinical application. Chin J Plastic Surg Burns 1991;7:8–10.

12. Hyakusoku H, Gao JH. The "super-thin" flap. Br J Plast Surg 1994;47(7):457–64.

13. Kwon JG, Brown E, Suh HP, et al. Planes for Perforator/Skin Flap Elevation-Definition, Classification, and Techniques. J Reconstr Microsurg 2023;39(3): 179–86.

14. Saint-Cyr M, Wong C, Schaverien M, et al. The perforasome theory: vascular anatomy and clinical implications. Plast Reconstr Surg 2009;124(05): 1529–44.

15. Giunta RE, Geisweid A, Feller AM. The value of preoperative Doppler sonography for planning free perforator flaps. Plast Reconstr Surg 2000;105: 2381–6.

16. Nahabedian MY. Overview of perforator imaging and flap perfusion technologies. Clin Plast Surg 2011;38(2):165–74.

17. Klein MB, Karanas YL, Chow LC, et al. Early experience with computed tomographic angiography in microsurgical reconstruction. Plast Reconstr Surg 2003;112(2):498–503.

18. Visconti G, Bianchi A, Hayashi A, et al. Thin and super-thin perforator flap elevation based on preoperative planning with ultrahigh-frequency ultrasound. Arch Plast Surg 2020;47(4):365–70.

19. Kimura N, Satoh K. Consideration of a thin flap as an entity and clinical applications of the thin anterolateral thigh flap. Plast Reconstr Surg 1996;97(5):985–92.

20. Yildirim S, Avci G, Aköz T. Soft-tissue reconstruction using a free anterolateral thigh flap: experience with 28 patients. Ann Plast Surg 2003;51(1):37–44.

21. Suh YC, Kim SH, Baek WY, et al. Super-thin ALT flap elevation using preoperative color doppler ultrasound planning: Identification of horizontally running pathway at the deep adipofascial layers. J Plast Reconstr Aesthetic Surg 2022;75(2):665–73.

22. Agostini T, Lazzeri D, Spinelli G. Anterolateral thigh flap thinning: techniques and complications. Ann Plast Surg 2014;72(2):246–52.

23. Kimura N, Satoh K, Hosaka Y. Microdissected thin perforator flaps: 46 cases. Plast Reconstr Surg 2003;112(7):1875–85.

24. Nojima K, Brown SA, Acikel C, et al. Defining vascular supply and territory of thinned perforator flaps: part I. Anterolateral thigh perforator flap. Plast Reconstr Surg 2005;116(1):182–93.

25. Cigna E, Minni A, Barbaro M, et al. An experience on primary thinning and secondary debulking of anterolateral thigh flap in head and neck reconstruction. Eur Rev Med Pharmacol Sci 2012; 16(8):1095–101.

26. Chang SC, Miller G, Halbert CF, et al. Limiting donor site morbidity by suprafascial dissection of the radial forearm flap. Microsurgery 1996;17(3):136–40.

27. Iida T, Mihara M, Yoshimatsu H, et al. Versatility of the superficial circumflex iliac artery perforator flap in head and neck reconstruction. Ann Plast Surg 2014;72(3):332–6.

28. Iida T, Yoshimatsu H, Tashiro K, et al. Reconstruction of a full-thickness, complex nasal defect that includes the nasal septum using a free, thin superficial inferior epigastric artery flap. Microsurgery 2016; 36(1):66–9.

29. Bali ZU, Karatan B, Parspanci A, et al. Total nasal reconstruction with pre-laminated, super-thin anterolateral thigh flap: A case report. Microsurgery 2021; 41(6):569–73.

30. Burget GC, Walton RL. Optimal use of microvascular free flaps, cartilage grafts, and a paramedian forehead flap for aesthetic reconstruction of the nose and adjacent facial units. Plast Reconstr Surg 2007;120(5):1171–207.

31. Cai YC, Li C, Zeng DF, et al. Comparative Analysis of Radial Forearm Free Flap and Anterolateral Thigh Flap in Tongue Reconstruction after Radical Resection of Tongue Cancer. ORL J Otorhinolaryngol Relat Spec 2019;81(5–6):252–64.

32. Webster HR, Robinson DW. The radial forearm flap without fascia and other refinements. Eur J Plast Surg 1995;18:11.

33. Chang SCN, Miller G, Halbert CF, et al. Limiting donor site morbidity by suprafascial dissection of the radial forearm flap. Microsurgery 1996;17:136.

34. Huang CH, Chen HC, Huang YL, et al. Comparison of the radial forearm flap and the thinned anterolateral

thigh cutaneous flap for reconstruction of tongue defects: an evaluation of donor-site morbidity. Plast Reconstr Surg 2004;114(7):1704–10.

35. Ma C, Tian Z, Kalfarentzos E, et al. Superficial circumflex iliac artery perforator flap for tongue reconstruction. Oral Surg Oral Med Oral Pathol Oral Radiol 2016;121(4):373–80.

36. Papanikolas MJ, Hurrell MJL, Clark JR, et al. Anterolateral thigh, radial forearm and superficial circumflex iliac perforator flaps in oral reconstruction: a comparative analysis. ANZ J Surg 2023;93(5): 1335–40.

37. Acartürk TO, Maldonado AA, Ereso A. Intraoral reconstruction with "thinned" peroneal artery perforator flaps: An alternative to classic donor areas in comorbid patients. Microsurgery 2015;35(5):399–402.

38. Ozkan O, Ozkan O, Coskunfirat OK, et al. Reconstruction of large palatal defects using the free anterolateral thigh flap. Ann Plast Surg 2011;66(6): 618–22.

39. Ooi ASH, Gill HS, Kiong KL, et al. Novel Endoscopic Transnasal Technique for Anterolateral Thigh Flap Inset Post Nasopharyngeal Carcinoma Resection. Plast Reconstr Surg Glob Open 2021; 9(7):e3665.

40. Yamamoto T, Yamamoto N, Ishiura R. Free double-paddle superficial circumflex iliac perforator flap transfer for partial maxillectomy reconstruction: A case report. Microsurgery 2022;42(1):84–8.

41. Narushima M, Yamasoba T, Iida T, et al. Pure skin perforator flap for microtia and congenital aural atresia using supermicrosurgical techniques. J Plast Reconstr Aesthetic Surg 2011;64(12): 1580–4.

42. Narushima M, Yamasoba T, Iida T, et al. Supermicrosurgical reconstruction for congenital aural atresia using a pure skin perforator flap: concept and long-term results. Plast Reconstr Surg 2013;131(6): 1359–66.

Customized Soft Tissue Free Flaps in Head and Neck Reconstruction

Susana Heredero, MD, PhD, FEBOMFS[a,b,]*,
Maria Isabel Falguera, MD, FEBOMFS[b], Vicenç Gómez, MD[c],
Alba Sanjuan-Sanjuan, MD, PhD[d]

KEYWORDS

- Microsurgery • Computed tomography angiography • Perforator mapping • Free flap
- Head and neck

KEY POINTS

- Advanced imaging technologies such as computed tomography angiography and color Doppler ultrasonography allow precise preoperative planning for soft tissue free flap reconstruction in head and neck surgery.
- Customization of flap selection, thickness, and design based on detailed mapping and study of perforator anatomy enhances surgical precision and minimizes intraoperative revisions.
- These technologies facilitate the harvesting of thinner and more sophisticated perforator flaps, expanding surgical options, reducing donor site morbidity, and improving functional and aesthetic results.
- Surgeon-led preoperative assessment using advanced imaging techniques reduces risks associated with anatomic vascular variations, such as partial or total flap loss, ensuring safer dissections and improved patient-specific results.

 Video content accompanies this article at http://www.oralmaxsurgery.theclinics.com.

INTRODUCTION

Over the past decade, computerized surgical planning (CSP) and computer-aided design and manufacturing (CAD/CAM) have seen exponential growth in bony free flap head and neck reconstruction. However, except for the use of computed tomography angiography (CTA) for preoperative planning of the deep inferior epigastric artery perforator (DIEP) flap—the current gold standard free flap for breast reconstruction—CSP for soft tissue free flaps is not as widely utilized, especially in head and neck reconstruction. Nevertheless, preoperative planning of soft tissue perforator free flaps with CTA and color Doppler ultrasonography (CDU) has gained popularity in recent years, thanks to ongoing technologies advancements.

Improvements in these technologies have also enabled the search for thinner and more sophisticated perforator flaps, allowing for better adaptation to the defects being reconstructed. This allows the

[a] Department of Maxillofacial Surgery, Hospital Universitario Reina Sofía, Avd. Menéndez Pidal s/n, Córdoba 14004, Spain; [b] Unidad de Cirugía Reconstructiva Avanzada, Hospital Cruz Roja, Paseo de la Victoria s/n, Córdoba 14004, Spain; [c] Department of Maxillofacial Surgery, Hospital Universitario Vall d'Hebron, Pg. Vall d'Hebron 119, Barcelona 08035, Spain; [d] Oral and Maxillofacial Surgery, Charleston Area Medical Center, Charleston, WV 24314, USA

* Corresponding author. Department of Maxillofacial Surgery, Hospital Universitario Reina Sofía, Avd. Menéndez Pidal s/n, Córdoba 14004, Spain.

E-mail address: susana_heredero@yahoo.es

Oral Maxillofacial Surg Clin N Am 36 (2024) 545–555
https://doi.org/10.1016/j.coms.2024.07.009

surgeon to customize flap selection, thickness, and design based on the specific characteristics of the vascular configuration and perforator anatomy in various possible donor sites for each individual.

In this article, we will review the accumulated knowledge that has enabled us to customize soft tissue free flaps in head and neck reconstruction and the current authors' approach.

HISTORICAL PERSPECTIVE

Perforator flaps have become workhorse flaps in soft tissue reconstruction, with those from the thigh being the most commonly used in head and neck procedures, especially the anterolateral (ALT) flap. The ALT flap was first described by Baek[1] and Song and colleagues[2] in the 80s. In 2002, Wei and colleagues[3] popularized it reporting the largest series to that date with 475 flaps for head and neck reconstruction. They also described the suprafascial elevation technique, which allowed the harvest of a thinner flap with less donor site morbidity by preserving the deep fascia. It was not until more than 10 years later that JP Hong hypothesized that by elevating the flap in the fascial layer between the deep and the superficial fat, the superficial fascia, they would be able to obtain an even thinner and hemodynamically reliable flap without unnecessary extra adipose tissue, avoiding the need for additional debulking procedures and improving the contour of the donor site.[4] Subsequently, this author demonstrated the effectiveness of this technique for the gluteal artery,[5,6] the superficial circumflex femoral artery[6,7] (SCIP), and the thoracodorsal artery perforator free flaps.[8] We have also demonstrated the feasibility of using the thin profunda artery perforator (PAP) flap as a valid option for tongue reconstruction.[9]

More recently, perforator flaps harvested in planes even more superficial to the superficial fascia layer have been described: superthin and pure skin perforator flaps, the latest ones including the dermal plexus without any superficial fat.[10] This evolution toward thinner flaps safely dissected in more superficial planes has been made possible thanks to advancements in various imaging technologies.

The use of CSP in bony free flap head and neck reconstruction, together with CAD/CAM, has been popularized in recent years. These technologies have also led to better outcomes in restoring function more efficiently. Various meta-analyses suggest that mandible reconstruction with a fibula osteocutaneous free flap using CSP and CAD/CAM is associated with shorter operating times, reduced ischemia time, more accurate and functional results, and greater cost-effectiveness compared to conventional techniques.[11–14] CSP planning has also

been implemented in soft tissue free flaps, especially the use of CTA for preoperative planning of the DIEP flap in breast reconstruction, as first described by Masià and colleagues, decreasing operative time and improving results.[15] CTA is considered the gold standard technique for the preoperative assessment of DIEP flaps; however, CDU has gained popularity recently and has become an increasingly attractive alternative.[16] Recently, Bajus and colleagues has conducted a randomized control trial showing that CDU mapping is equally effective as CTA combined with CDU in locating relevant perforators of the DIEP flap.[17]

Although the reported literature is much smaller, CSP and CTA have been used to assess perforator flaps other than the DIEP flap. Moreover, Chim and colleagues used CTA not only for perforator mapping but also to characterize perforator anatomy in the subcutaneous tissue in the PAP flap. They used this knowledge to safely elevate thin flaps for limbs reconstruction.[18–20] Similarly, Visconti and colleagues reported their experience using CDU with ultra-high frequencies to better assess the subcutaneous tissue's perforator anatomy in both ALT and SCIP flaps.[21,22]

The free-style elevation of perforator flaps was first described by Mardini and Wei in 2003.[23] In their technique description, superficial flaps dissected above the deep fascia were designed around a pre-identified sizable skin vessel using Doppler signals and an exploratory incision. They noted that the main disadvantage of free-style free flaps was the possibility of inaccurately mapping the skin vessel, and the inability to predict preoperatively the size of the vessels and the pedicle length. However, advancements in perforator imaging technology over the last 2 decades have addressed these issues. Additionally, detailed information on the anatomy of vessels within the subcutaneous tissue nowadays allows for better assessment and selection of potential donor sites, enabling safer harvest of thin and superthin flaps.

NATURE OF THE PROBLEM

Soft tissue reconstruction in the head and neck area presents significant challenges due to the diverse range of defects, each with its own functional and aesthetic considerations. Depending on the reconstruction site, we may require a skin island with different characteristics such as specific area, thickness, pliability, or additional tissue components. Traditionally, flap selection has been based on the general characteristics of the various donor sites. For instance, the radial forearm free flap (RFFF) is generally the preferable choice worldwide for hemiglossectomy reconstruction when a thin and pliable flap is required.[24] The truth is there is no other free flap available in the body that reunites the same combination of thickness, pliability and pedicle length as the RFFF. However, advancements in dissection techniques that enable the safe harvesting of thinner or variable-thickness flaps have broadened the application of certain flaps in head and neck reconstruction. Previously deemed too bulky, these flaps are now viable options, particularly in Western populations, such as the PAP flap (**Figs. 1** and **2**).

If thin flaps harvested from the plane of the superficial fascia layer are not yet widely adopted in head and neck reconstructive surgery, even thinner flaps are less commonly used. The main drawbacks are the difficulty in mastering the dissection technique and the limitations in utilizing the CSP and the most advanced imaging technologies.

CSP with CTA can be challenging for several reasons. First, identifying the anatomy of the perforator within the subcutaneous tissue is difficult, especially when there is a thin layer of fat. It has been shown that administration of sublingual nitroglycerin before CTA dilates small peripheral arteries,

increases the number of evaluable branches, and delineates the relationship of septal or muscle branches with perforators more clearly.[25] Additionally, we have described our technique using the open-source software HorosTM, v 3.3.6 (GNU Lesser General Public License, version 3) for data postprocessing.[26] This software has a tool named maximum intensity projection, which allows the voxel to be projected with the highest attenuation value on every view throughout the volume onto a 2 dimension image by combining different CTA sections, making small vessels visible. Furthermore, translating the data gathered from the CTA to the patient in the operating room can be done in various ways: using CTA measurements and traditional anatomic landmarks, handheld Doppler, CDU, or mixed reality (MR)/augmented reality (AR) technologies.[27]

Nowadays, many surgeons advocate for the use of CDU over CTA for preoperative planning of soft tissue free flaps. The advantages and disadvantages of both techniques are summarized in **Table 1**. While CDU offers easier availability and data transfer to the patient, CTA allows for

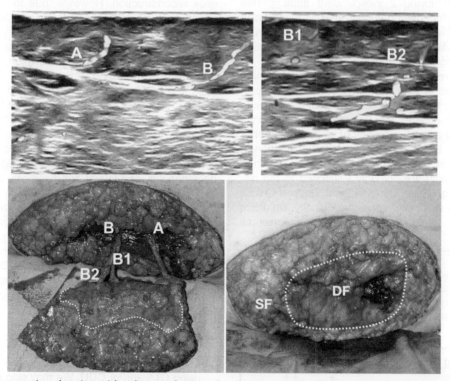

Fig. 1. Preoperative planning with color coppler Doppler ultrasonography (CDU) and intraoperative images of a dissected customized thickness profunda artery perforator (PAP) flap and its donor site. This flap includes a peripheral area dissected above the plane of the superficial fascia layer (white dotted line) and a thicker part around both perforators dissected in the plane of the superficial fascia layer. A: proximal perforator; B: distal perforator, divided into two branches; B1: proximal branch of the distal perforator; B2: distal branch of the distal perforator; SF: superficial fat; DF: deep fat.

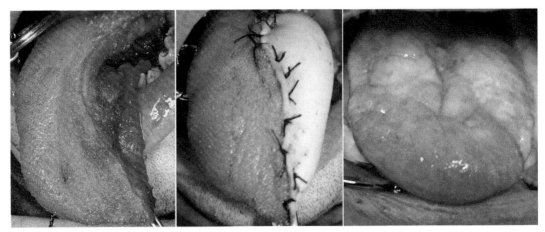

Fig. 2. Hemiglossectomy reconstruction with a customized thickness PAP flap, immediate and 5-year postoperative reconstructions.

better evaluation of deeper anatomic structures and quicker assessment of all potential donor sites in the lower limbs. Therefore, CTA is particularly valuable in assessing vascular anatomic variations, such as the feasibility of harvesting a chimeric PAP-gracilis flap from a common pedicle versus employing 2 independent flaps.[28] This approach has been demonstrated as a good and straightforward option for dynamic reconstruction, utilizing 2 flaps (chimeric or independent) from a single donor site in a single stage.[29]

Our current approach for preoperative planning of soft tissue free flaps involves CTA, supplemented by the prior administration of nitroglycerin (except for patients with formal contraindications), to provide a quick overview of all potential donor sites. This is followed by a detailed evaluation of the optimal options using CDU. Data obtained from planning are primarily translated to the patient using CDU, with handheld Doppler (HHD) remaining as an alternative. Additionally, we utilize MR/AR in selected cases where 3-dimensional

(3D) assessment is crucial or for educational purposes among junior surgeons.[27]

PROCEDURAL APPROACH

Several soft tissue flaps can be used for head and neck reconstruction. However, due to considerations such as both the 2-team approach and the lower donor site morbidity, our preferred choices are those harvested from the lower limbs, including the ALT, the anteromedial thigh, the PAP, the medial sural artery perforator, and the SCIP flaps. The RFFF, although offering an ideal combination of thickness, pliability, and pedicle length, is our second option due to its proximity to the resection area and higher donor site morbidity. Furthermore, other flaps, such as the thoracodorsal artery perforator, latissimus dorsi, scapular and parascapular, and lateral arm flaps are also near the resection area and are not our primary options. However, these flaps harvested from donor sites different from the lower limbs can be considered as alternatives for patients experiencing recurrences or complications requiring secondary reconstructions, as well as for complex 3D defects or patients with insufficient recipient vessels near the reconstruction site and longer pedicle lengths are needed.

Considering this, our workflow for flap selection and design is as follows.

1. In general, we do preoperative assessments using CTA and/or CDU. We may skip this step only if we know from the beginning that the selected flap will be dissected just above or below the deep fascia. However, additional advantages of preoperative assessment in these cases will also be discussed later.

Table 1
Comparison between color Doppler ultrasonography (CDU) and computed tomography angiography (CTA) for perforator flap assessment

	CDU	CTA
Learning curve	+++	++
Price	+	++
Morbidity	NO	YES
Data transfer to the patient	EASY	DIFFICULT
Depth	LOW	HIGH
Assessment time	+++	+

Table 2
Characteristics of flaps

	RF/UF	LA	ALT/AMT	SCIP	MSAP	PAP
Thickness	+	++	+++	+	++	++++
Pliability	++++	++	++	++++	++	++++
Pedicle length	++++	++	+++	+	++	++
Donor site morbidity	+++	+++	++	+	++	+

Abbreviations: ALT, anterolateral thigh; AMT, anteromedial thigh; LA, lateral arm; MSAP, medial sural artery perforator; PAP, profunda artery perforator; RF, radial forearm; SCIP, superficial circumflex iliac artery perforator; UF, ulnar forearm

2. Next, we evaluate which flap would be the best for the defect, considering the intrinsic characteristics of the different flaps such as thickness, pliability, pedicle length, and donor site morbidity (**Table 2**).
3. Finally, we evaluate which flap is the best for the specific patient. This decision is essential when the defect needs to be reconstructed with thin and/or superthin flaps, and it is made after studying the anatomy of the perforators in each location, mainly within the subcutaneous tissue. This information can be assessed with either CTA or CDU and will allow us to tailor a flap that ensures the preservation of an adequate vascular flow (**Fig. 3**).

OUTCOMES

We applied this workflow to customize flap selection, thickness, and design in 20 consecutive patients (the virtual surgical planning [VSP] group). We compared them to a group of 22 consecutive patients whose flap selection and design did not follow this workflow (the non-VSP group). 2 independent reconstructive teams led and performed surgery in each group of patients, following these 2 different approaches. All patients' data are summarized in **Table 3**.

In the VSP group, the surgeon (first author of this article) conducted data postprocessing of the preoperative CTA to assess perforator location and anatomy. This information was then integrated into the operating room using CDU, MR/AR, or HHD. Consequently, the design of the skin island primarily relied on preoperative assessment rather than traditional anatomic landmarks.

Conversely, in the non-VSP group, data postprocessing were performed by the radiologist, who provided information solely on perforator mapping without detailing perforator anatomy.

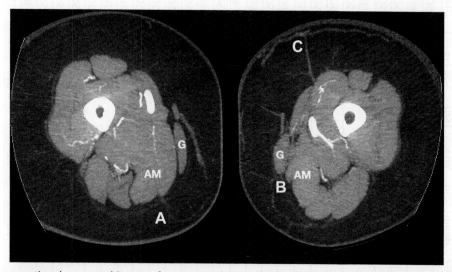

Fig. 3. Cross-sectional processed image of a computed tomography angiography (CTA) using HorosTM, v 3.3.6 (GNU Lesser General Public License, version 3) and the maximum intensity projection software tool showing 3 perforators. Perforators A and C correspond to the PAP flap area, whereas perforator B is in the anteromedial thigh flap area. Both perforators A and C are divided close to the cutaneous surface, making it easier to harvest a thin or superthin flap. However, perforator B is divided into branches near the deep fascia.

Table 3
Data related to the patient's cohort included for evaluating our workflow in customizing flap selection, thickness and design

#	Gender	Height (cm)	Weight (Kg)	Age (years)	Diagnosis	Location	Flap	Plane	VSP Group	TNG
1	M	160	70	73,3	SSC	Tongue	SCIP	Thin	Yes	No
2	M	180	68	59	Secondary	FOM	SCIP	Thin	Yes	No
3	M	158	71	68,9	SSC	Tongue	SCIP	Thin	Yes	No
4	F	153	45	76	SSC	Tongue	ALT	Thin	Yes	No
5	F	159	82	75,5	Estesioneuroblastoma	Skull Base	ALT	Thin	Yes	No
6	M	176	77	59	SSC	FOM	ALT	Thin	Yes	No
7	M	170	108	59,7	SSC	FOM	ALT	Suprafascial	No	No
8	F	162	70	85,1	SSC	Retromolar Trigone	PAP	Subfascial	No	No
9	M	172	79	66,4	SSC	Retromolar Trigone	PAP	Subfascial	No	No
10	M	172	75	61,9	Secondary	SCALP	SCIP	Thin	Yes	No
11	M	166	68	61,9	SSC	Tongue	ALT	Suprafascial	No	No
12	M	165	71	60,3	SSC	Tongue	PAP	Thin	Yes	No
13	M	176	100	46,7	Meningioma	Skull Base	PAP	Thin	Yes	No
14	M	162	70,5	83,7	BSC	Nose	SCIP	Thin	Yes	No
15	F	151	48	78,6	Secondary	Lower Face	ALT	Thin	Yes	No
16	M	184	85	57,3	SSC	FOM	ALT	Suprafascial	No	No
17	F	149	82	71,9	SSC	Alveolar Ridge	ALT	Suprafascial	No	No
18	F	143	47	80,2	SSC	Buccal	ALT	Suprafascial	No	No
19	F	165	55	58,2	SSC	Oropharynx	PAP	Subfascial	No	Yes
20	M	180	100	54,9	Meningioma	SCALP	ALT	Thin	Yes	No
21	M	178	87	56,5	SSC	Oropharynx	PAP	Suprafascial	Yes	No
22	M	178	87	69	SSC	FOM	ALT	Suprafascial	No	No
23	M	171	85	37,5	SSC	Tongue	ALT	Suprafascial	No	No
24	M	178	130	69	SSC	Tongue	PAP (gracilis)	Chimeric	No	Yes
25	F	158	80	68,3	SSC	Tongue	ALT	Suprafascial	No	Yes
26	M	166	77	68,3	BSC	Cheek - nose	ALT	Suprafascial	No	No
27	F	162	55	59	SSTR	SCALP	AMT	Thin	Yes	No
28	F	154	56	56,3	SSC	Tongue	ALT	Subfascial	No	No
29	F	157	66	67,7	Glioblastoma	Scalp	PAP	Thin	Yes	No

30	M	172	93	48	Meningioma	SCALP	ALT	Suprafascial	Yes	No
31	F	160	62	48	SSC	Tongue	SCIP	Thin	Yes	No
32	M	161	75	47,8	SSTR	Neck	ALT	Suprafascial	No	No
33	M	158	65	76,7	SSC	Alveolar Ridge	ALT	Suprafascial	No	Yes
34	M	173	87	69,8	SSC	Alveolar Ridge	ALT	Subfascial	No	No
35	M	155	70,5	69,9	SSC	Cervical recurrence	ALT	Subfascial	No	No
36	F	145	57	67,7	SSC	Tongue	ALT	Thin	Yes	No
37	M	178	81	49	SSC	Tongue	ALT	Thin	Yes	No
38	F	145	50	65,5	SSC	Tongue	ALT	Suprafascial	No	No
39	M	172	74	69,9	SSC	Tongue	ALT	Suprafascial	No	No
40	F	151	54	65,4	SSC	Tongue	ALT	Suprafascial	No	No
41	M	165	72	76,8	SSC	Alveolar ridge	ALT	Suprafascial	No	No
42	F	155	45	15	SSTR	Submental	ALT	Suprafascial	Yes	No

Abbreviations: ALT, anterolateral thigh; AMT, anteromedial thigh; FOM, floor of the mouth; PAP, profunda artery perforator; SCIP, superficial circumflex iliac artery perforator; SSC, squamous cell carcinoma; SSTR, secondary soft tissue reconstruction; TNG, the need to change the preoperative flap design; VSP, virtual surgical planning.

This information was conveyed to the surgical team using traditional anatomic landmarks and HHD.

The VSP group included 9 ALT, 4 PAP, 6 SCIP, and 1 AMT flap. All were thin flaps dissected above the superficial fascial layer, except for 3 flaps dissected just above the deep fascia (2 ALT and 1 PAP flap). In the non-VSP group, 18 ALT flaps and 4 PAP flaps were planned, although one of the flaps initially intended as a PAP flap was finally harvested as a gracilis myocutaneous flap.

The main variable comparing these 2 cohorts was "the need to change the preoperative flap design." There was no need to change the initial flap design in any of the flaps of the VSP group, whereas it had to be changed in 4 flaps of the non-VSP group.

The skin island of the flap design in case #19 needed to be changed to include 2 perforators that did not pierce the skin where predicted.

In case #24, the initial design was based on anatomic indications by the radiologist for a PAP flap. However, the non-VSP surgical team had to switch to a gracilis myocutaneous flap because the PAP perforators were not adequately mapped. Subsequent evaluation of the patient's CTA revealed that the main PAP perforator was located more posteriorly in the thigh than described by the radiologist (**Fig. 4**). Similarly, in clinical case #33, the initial flap design was based on information provided by the radiologist regarding to 2 existing perforators in the ALT area. However, during surgery, it was found that these vessels, identified by the non-VSP team with that information in the radiological report and HHD, were instead tensor fascia lata perforator and another vessel originating from the

AMT area. This vessel followed a long lateral trajectory within the subcutaneous tissue before reaching the skin. We could observe this discrepancy postoperatively using our workflow for data processing, as described earlier (Videos 1 and 2). Radiologists may not be familiar with the anatomic variations of perforators and can inadvertently convey incorrect information to the surgeon. This highlights the importance of the preoperative study being conducted by the surgeons themselves.

The last case in which the non-VSP group required a change in the initial flap design is case #25. The flap was originally designed based on a septocutaneous vessel in the ALT region. However, after piercing the deep fascia, it followed a long lateral longitudinal trajectory and pierced the skin more laterally than anticipated. As a result, surgeons had to reposition the skin island to the lateral thigh.

On the other hand, within the VSP group, the application of our workflow proved valuable in preventing the need to change the initial flap design and mitigating potential complications, such as those expected with thin flaps, for reasons detailed earlier in this article. Moreover, we have found it beneficial in preventing complications, even with cutaneous flaps that include a substantial amount of subcutaneous tissue. For instance, in clinical case #20, a patient was reconstructed with an ALT flap based on a perforator that, after penetrating the deep fascia, followed a long longitudinal course within the subcutaneous tissue before dividing into 2 branches and piercing the skin laterally (see Video 3 and **Fig. 5**). Although, as mentioned in the procedural approach section of this article, preoperative planning may be considered unnecessary when

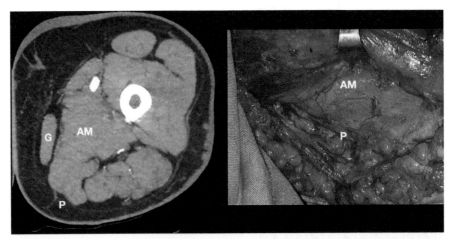

Fig. 4. CTA and intraoperative image of the donor site after harvesting a gracilis myocutaneous flap showing an adductor magnus perforator in the posteromedial thigh, piercing the skin posteriorly. AM, adductor magnus muscle; G, gracilis muscle; P, adductor magnus perforator.

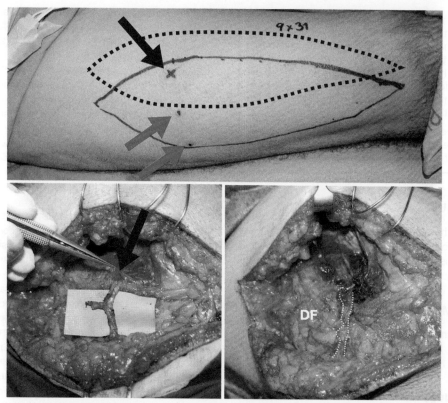

Fig. 5. Anterolateral thigh flap designed based on previous preoperative imaging. The "x" and the black arrow indicate the point where the perforator pierces the deep fascia. Red arrows indicate the points where its branches reach the skin. The black dotted line represents where the skin island would have been designed if only traditional anatomic landmarks and the point where the perforator was most audible with handheld Doppler were considered. The dotted white line outlines the longitudinal lateral trajectory of the perforator within the subcutaneous tissue. DF, deep fat lobules.

harvesting a flap just above or below the deep fascia, the lateral trajectory within the subcutaneous tissue encountered can only be identified through preoperative imaging.

SUMMARY

Expanding our armamentarium by customizing the selection, thickness, and design of our flaps can help us better adapt them to specific defects. We can now evaluate all the available perforators for different flap options and customize them. Using preoperative soft tissue planning, we have the ability to modify the area and volume of the skin island, add multiple skin paddles, incorporate other tissue components in a chimeric fashion, predict pedicle length, know possible anatomic vascular variations, and design flaps based on the anatomy of the perforator within the subcutaneous tissue. Knowing this information beforehand helps us select the best donor site and ensures safer dissections.

CLINICS CARE POINTS

- Customizing soft tissue perforator flap selection, thickness, and design can be safely achieved using various preoperative imaging modalities, such as CDU and CTA.

- While CDU offers lower morbidity, reduced cost, and facilitates data transfer in the operating room, CTA allows for quicker and more comprehensive evaluation of potential donor sites and assessment of deeper anatomic structures.

- Preoperative planning for soft tissue free flaps has proven beneficial not only for mapping and selecting the most suitable perforator, as seen with the DIEP flap over recent decades, and for perforator flaps from the lower limbs. This planning facilitates understanding of perforator anatomy within the subcutaneous tissue, enabling safer dissection of thinner flaps.

- Long trajectories of perforators within the subcutaneous tissue before reaching the skin may be observed, particularly in patients with thicker subcutaneous tissue or those with higher body mass indexes who have experienced weight loss. However, this phenomenon can also occur in patients who do not fit these conditions.
- Preoperative assessment must be conducted by the surgeons themselves to minimize the risk of complications.

DISCLOSURES

None of the authors has a financial interest in any of the products, devices, or drugs mentioned in this manuscript. The study was not financially supported by any grants.

SUPPLEMENTARY DATA

Supplementary data to this article can be found online at https://doi.org/10.1016/j.coms.2024.07.009.

REFERENCES

1. Baek SM. Two new cutaneous free flaps: the medial and lateral thigh flaps. Plast Reconstr Surg 1983;71: 354–65.
2. Song YG, Chen GZ, Song YL. The free thigh flap: a new free flap concept based on the septocutaneous artery. Br J Plast Surg 1984;37:149–59.
3. Wei FC, Jain V, Celik N, et al. Have we found an ideal soft-tissue flap? An experience with 672 anterolateral thigh flaps. Plast Reconstr Surg 2002;109: 2219–26 [discussion 2227-2230].
4. Hong JP, Chung IW. The superficial fascia as a new plane of elevation for anterolateral thigh flaps. Ann Plast Surg 2013;70(2):192–5.
5. Hong JP, Yim JH, Malzone G, et al. The thin gluteal artery perforator free flap to resurface the posterior aspect of the leg and foot. Plast Reconstr Surg 2014;133(5):1184–91.
6. Hong JP, Choi DH, Suh H, et al. A new plane of elevation: the superficial fascial plane for perforator flap elevation. J Reconstr Microsurg 2014;30(7):491–6. Epub 2014 Feb 19.
7. Goh TLH, Park SW, Cho JY, et al. The search for the ideal thin skin flap: superficial circumflex iliac artery perforator flap–a review of 210 cases. Plast Reconstr Surg 2015;135(2):592–601.
8. Kim KN, Hong JP, Park CR, et al. Modification of the elevation plane and defatting technique to create a thin thoracodorsal artery perforator flap. J Reconstr Microsurg 2016;32(2):142–6. Epub 2015 Aug 31.
9. Heredero S, Sanjuan A, Falguera MI, et al. The thin profunda femoral artery perforator flap for tongue reconstruction. Microsurgery 2020;40(2):117–24. Epub 2019 Jun 24.PMID: 31233631.
10. Yamamoto T, Yamamoto N, Fuse Y, et al. Subdermal dissection for elevation of pure skin perforator flaps and superthin flaps: the dermis as a landmark for the most superficial dissection plane. Plast Reconstr Surg 2021;147(3):470–8.
11. Pucci R, Weyh A, Smotherman C, et al. Accuracy of virtual planned surgery versus conventional freehand surgery for reconstruction of the mandible with osteocutaneous free flaps. Int J Oral Maxillofac Surg 2020;49(9):1153–61.
12. Padilla PL, Mericli AF, Largo RD, et al. Computeraided design and manufacturing versus conventional surgical planning for head and neck reconstruction: a systematic review and meta-analysis. Plast Reconstr Surg 2021;148(1):183–92.
13. Salinero L, Boczar D, Barrow B, et al. Patient-centred outcomes and dental implant placement in computer-aided free flap mandibular reconstruction: a systematic review and meta-analysis. Br J Oral Maxillofac Surg 2022;60(10):1283–91. Epub 2022 Sep 28.
14. Kurlander DE, Garvey PB, Largo RD, et al. The cost utility of virtual surgical planning and computerassisted design/computer-assisted manufacturing in mandible reconstruction using the free fibula osteocutaneous flap. J Reconstr Microsurg 2023;39(3): 221–30.
15. Masia J, Clavero JA, Larrañaga JR, et al. Multidetector-row computed tomography in the planning of abdominal perforator flaps. J Plast Reconstr Aesthetic Surg 2006;59(6):594–9.
16. Perez-Iglesias CT, Laikhter E, Kang CO, et al. Current applications of ultrasound imaging in the preoperative planning of DIEP Flaps. J Reconstr Microsurg 2022;38(3):221–7. Epub 2022 Jan 28.
17. Bajus A, Streit L, Kubek T, et al. Color Doppler ultrasound versus CT angiography for DIEP flap planning: A randomized controlled trial. Plast Reconstr Aesthet Surg 2023;86:48–57. Epub 2023 Jul 23.
18. Chim H. The superthin profunda artery perforator flap for extremity reconstruction: clinical implications. Plast Reconstr Surg 2022;150(4):915–8.
19. Chim H. Suprafascial radiological characteristics of the superthin profunda artery perforator flap. J Plast Reconstr Aesthetic Surg 2022;75(7):2064–9.
20. Chim H. Perforator mapping and clinical experience with the superthin profunda artery perforator flap for reconstruction in the upper and lower extremities. J Plast Reconstr Aesthetic Surg 2023;81:60–7.
21. Visconti G, Bianchi A, Hayashi A, et al. Thin and superthin perforator flap elevation based on preoperative planning with ultrahigh-frequency ultrasound. Arch Plast Surg 2020;47(4):365–70. Epub 2020 Jul 15.

22. Visconti G, Bianchi A, Hayashi A, et al. Designing an anterolateral thigh flap using ultrasound. J Reconstr Microsurg 2022;38(3):206–16. Epub 2021 Dec 17.

23. Mardini S, Tsai FC, Wei FC. The thigh as a model for free style free flaps. Clin Plast Surg 2003;30(3):473–80.

24. Kansy K, Mueller AA, Mücke T, et al. A worldwide comparison of the management of T1 and T2 anterior floor of the mouth and tongue squamous cell carcinoma - Extent of surgical resection and reconstructive measures. J Cranio-Maxillo-Fac Surg 2017;45(12):2097–104. Epub 2017 Sep 21.

25. Watanabe M, Murakami R, Miyauchi R, et al. Utility of preoperative multidetector-row computed tomographic angiography after sublingual nitroglycerin with three-dimensional reconstruction in planning of the anterolateral thigh flap. Plast Reconstr Surg 2020;145(2):407e–11e. PMID: 3198565.

26. Heredero S, Falguera-Uceda MI, Sanjuan-Sanjuan A, et al. Virtual planning of profunda femoral artery and superficial circumflex iliac artery perforator flaps. Plast Reconstr Surg Glob Open 2021;9(6):e3617.

27. Heredero S, Falguera MI, Marín A, et al. Virtual planning and mixed reality for the thin anterolateral thigh perforator flap. Plast Reconstr Surg Glob Open 2022;10(10):e4567.

28. Heredero S, Falguera-Uceda MI, Sanjuan-Sanjuan A, et al. Chimeric profunda artery perforator - gracilis flap: A computed tomographic angiography study and case report. Microsurgery 2021;41(3):250–7.

29. Yao CMK, Jozaghi Y, Danker S, et al. The combined profunda artery perforator-gracilis flap for immediate facial reanimation and resurfacing of the radical parotidectomy defect. Microsurgery 2023;43(4):309–15. Epub 2022 Dec 21.

Perforator Flaps and Robotic Surgery for Head and Neck Reconstruction

Francesco M.G. Riva, MD, FRCS*,
Cyrus Kerawala, FDSRCS, FRCS (OMFS), RCPathME

KEYWORDS

- Head and neck • Free flaps • Perforator flaps • Robotic surgery • Head and neck reconstruction
- Microvascular • Oropharyngeal squamous cell carcinoma

KEY POINTS

- Indications and contraindications for perforator free flap reconstruction with Transoral Robotic Surgery.
- Understanding indications for Transoral robotic Free Flap reconstruction.
- Understanding contraindications for Transoral Robotic Free Flap reconstruction.
- Introducing some refinements that help with some challenging steps of the procedure.

BACKGROUND

Head and neck cancer (HNC) is the sixth most common cancer across the world. Despite a general reduction in tobacco consumption and therefore reduction in risk exposure there has been an increasing incidence of oropharyngeal squamous cell carcinoma (OPSCC).[1]

This has been often linked to human papillomavirus (HPV). Patients in this cohort tend to be younger and generally present with a more favourable prognosis.[2]

Historically first line treatment for HPV-related OPSCC is chemo radiotherapy (CRT) to the head and neck area but this carries long term morbidity and considerable risk for conditions like osteoradionecrosis, whose incidence varies between 2% and 12% and can be highly debilitating, not infrequently requiring major surgery.[3]

It is important to understand that OPSCC not only threaten a patient's life, but even following traditional treatments they can have, long term, a great impact on the patient's appearance and physiologic function.[4]

HPV-related cancers of the head and neck are more sensitive to CRT but the longer survival draws more attention to the long-term side effects of non-surgical treatment.[5]

This has generated a drive to try and deescalate the morbidity of radiotherapy replacing it with surgery in selected cases.[6]

At the same time, despite primary treatments, there is rate of recurrence for OPSCC cancer of 17.3% versus 32.5% (P<.001) respectively for HPV+ and HPV- which needs to be taken into account.[7]

In the advanced cancer patients cohort, some 60% will develop recurrence, mostly loco regional.[8]

When feasible, salvage surgery is the standard of practice and historically vast majority of times it involves open surgery and some form of reconstruction with free tissue transfer.

Open surgery traditionally requires a lower lip split and a mandibulotomy for access, followed by wide local excision, and inevitably leaves visible scars through the neck and the chin, which may impact on speech and swallowing function,

Head and Neck Unit, The Royal Marsden NHS Foundation Trust, Fulham Road, London SW3 6JJ, UK
* Corresponding author.
E-mail address: francesco.riva@rmh.nhs.uk

Oral Maxillofacial Surg Clin N Am 36 (2024) 557–566
https://doi.org/10.1016/j.coms.2024.07.006

besides having a psychological impact on patients' quality of life.[4]

Given the above, it is easy to understand how more attention has shifted to minimal or less invasive surgical options with a drive from both patients and clinicians to try and reduce morbidity in the treatment of HNC, both limiting and avoiding the use of CRT and open surgery. Robotic surgery is naturally gaining momentum and support in this direction.[9,10]

O'Malley and colleagues[11] first introduced transoral robotic surgery (TORS) for treatment of cancers of the base of tongue in 2006.

Several studies since have shown the efficacy and safety of robotic surgery for cancers of the head and neck.[12,13,14]

In 2009 the use of the Da Vinci surgical system (Intuitive Surgical, Inc.–Sunnyvale CA) was approved by the United States Food and Drug Administration for the treatment of early-stage oropharyngeal tumors (T1/T2).

In 2010 Selber[15] first published a case series of oropharyngeal defects transorally reconstructed with the support of a robot.

Improvement in devices and skills have made transoral surgery more competitive and recently published multidisciplinary guidelines in the UK suggest that, in carefully selected patients, transoral surgery appears to be an effective alternative to open surgery for the management of recurrent OPSCC.[16]

More recently, Paleri and colleagues evaluated 26 patients considered potential candidates for TORS in salvage OPSCC. Of these, 21 underwent TORS and 5 open resection (4 due to unsuitable anatomy or tumor extension). At 42.6 months of follow-up, overall survival (OS) was 48.2%, with local control and disease-specific survival rates of 76.6% and 77.1%, respectively. Based on those findings, the authors concluded that TORS is a valid management option for residual and recurrent OPSCC. They also noted that oncologic outcomes were comparable to open surgery and translaser microsurgery, with the added advantage of en bloc resection, the ability to perform intraoperative ultrasound imaging, and to inset free flaps without mandibular split.[17]

We are looking at a cohort of patients who require top expertise in 2 fields: free tissue transfer and robotic transoral surgery.

Benefits of Transoral Robotic Surgery

Although Da Vinci (Intuitive Inc., Sunnyvale CA) has been one of the pioneers, several companies like Intuitive, CMR Surgical and Medtronic have now products available with slightly different features. All provide.

- Improved visualisation, especially in confined and narrow space
- 3-dimensional high resolution and high magnification
- Reduction of tremor
- Enhanced dexterity with 6° of freedom

In the field of oropharyngeal recurrent tumors, TORS offers an alternative surgical approach with acceptable oncologic and better functional outcomes than traditional open surgical approaches. This adds to the growing amount of clinical evidence to support the use of TORS in selected patients with recurrent oropharyngeal SCC as a feasible and oncologically sound method of treatment.[18]

Patients who underwent TORS were shown to have significantly improved outcomes in speech and swallowing function compared with those undergoing open surgery.

The TORS cases in our study had on average 6.7 times less blood loss.[18]

In a retrospective analysis comparing open surgery with TORS for recurrent OPSCC 30 patients were examined, 15 undergoing TORS and 15 an open approach.

The mean length of hospital stay was 35.2 days (range, 26–45 days) for those undergoing open surgery, compared to 19 days (range, 13–25 days) for those undergoing TORS (P<.001). Complications occurred in 6 patients (40%) with the open approach (haemorrhage in 2, pharyngocutaneous fistula in 2, and flap necrosis in 2) and in 4 patients (26.6%) in the TORS group (flap necrosis in 3 and cervical hematoma in 1; P=.01).[19]

TORS group had fewer complications (P=.01), better functional results (P=.003), and shorter surgical time (P<.001).[20]

Patients undergoing robotic surgery showed better results than the radical open surgery group in several areas deeply involved in quality-of-life evaluation, such as: pain, activity, recreation, swallowing, speech, anxiety.[21,22]

As oncologic treatments are getting better at local and regional control, and as part of a natural evolution in patients education and self-awareness the focus has widened from survival to quality of life and cosmesis.

In the past 2 decades there has been an increasing interest in minimally-invasive procedures as a mean to improve post treatment quality of life.

Survival from a cancer diagnosis has slowly evolved into quality of life after cancer treatment.

In the head and neck field there has been a lot of work done investigating scar perception from the patients' point of view in thyroid surgery.

The negative impact of scars is often underestimated by clinicians and most patients would choose to avoid a neck scar if given the option.

Indications for Free Flap after Transoral Robotic Surgery

Following TORS not all cases require reconstruction with free flap, although it becomes more and more important in the salvage setting, due to long term radiotherapy damage and delayed healing, to provide fresh healthy tissue with a free flap transfer.

Generally speaking, the main objectives of reconstruction in these cases are to.

- Cover critical structures such as major blood vessels
- Separate the oropharynx from the neck, achieving watertight seal
- Reduce velopharyngeal insufficiency; and
- Restore tongue volume and mobility.[23–25]

As a simple playbook rule we can say that free tissue transfer is required when.

- More than 1 anatomic subset is involved (tonsil, tongue base, soft palate, pharyngeal wall)
- Adverse features are present:
  ○ Carotid artery exposed
  ○ Through and through defects—more than 50% soft palate defect
  ○ Surgery is of a salvage nature (recurrent or persistent disease).[24]

Indications for Robotic Assisted Free Flap

Within the cohort of patients requiring a free flap following TORS as outlined above, the indications for a robotic-assisted inset may be limited to particularly challenging cases only.

Specifically, considering again the above-mentioned indications for free flap reconstruction, a robotic assisted free flap (RAFFI) may be limited to cases where multiple anatomic subsets are involved and, generally, all of the salvage cases.

A simple reconstruction of a lateral pharyngeal wall to cover major blood vessels most likely does not require robotic assistance. It can often be done transorally, unless trismus co-exists, which falls again into the salvage cohort.

Choice of Free Flap/Benefits of a Perforator Flap

Historically the first free flaps inset with the support of a robot were radial forearm free flaps because they have less bulk, which facilitates inset.

Radial forearm free flap has been for many years a fundamental tool of head and neck reconstruction, due to reliably think and pliable skin paddle, easy and relatively quick to harvest.

There are some inherent limitations though, such as:

- The need for a skin graft to repair the donor site, which carried longer healing time and much more scaring and in a more conspicuous area of the body.
- Tendon exposure as a not infrequent complication.
- Sacrifice of a major terminal vesse.l

In recent years the introduction of perforator flaps in the head and neck has increased the sophistication and the options available, offering more versatility.[26]

Since the first introduction of perforator free flaps by Koshima in 1989[27] and Song in 1984[28] flaps such Antero Lateral Thigh (ALT) have become a real workhorse for head and neck reconstruction and have become extremely popular in the microsurgical reconstructive community.[29–31]

The options of perforator flaps now available includes ALT flap, the real workhorse probably,[32] Thoraco Dorsal Artery Perforator Fflap, Medial Sural Artery Perforator (MSAP) flap, Antero Medial Thigh flap, Profunda Artery Perforator flap and Deep Inferior Epigastric Artery Perforator flap.[33]

When we look at reconstruction following transoral robotic though, choices are somehow more restricted.

As mentioned before we are looking at mostly salvage cases, following previous radiotherapy and sometimes surgery as well and we are looking at multiple anatomic subunits.

Keeping this in mind we understand the importance of

- Longer pedicle
- Potential for multiple perforators
- Potential for chimeric flap with muscle compound
- Potential to thin certain areas of the flap while maintaining bulk in others

The flap of choice becomes the ALT which, we due exceptions, ticks all the above boxes, being a flexible and robust reconstructive option while providing a tailored and targeted reconstruction.

- Described with a reliable pedicle length of 8 cm to 16 cm,[34] an ALT can almost certainly be always harvested with at least 12 cm of pedicle, which becomes very helpful in case of a depleted neck following previous treatment.

- A chimeric flap with a compound of vastus lateralis can be easily added to fill dead space or provide more bulk (**Fig. 1**).
- A solid fascia can be harvested and used as a second layer or as an anchor point when more support is needed, for example, on posterior and lateral pharyngeal wall.
- Separate skin paddles can be harvested using different perforators when the 3-dimensional complexity of the defect requires it. It is easy to understand this concept when we visualise a defect extending into pharyngeal wall, tongue base and soft palate.
- Tailoring the thickness of the flap to the area to reconstruct is extremely important and the ALT has been widely proved to be reliable and safe also as a thin to super thin flap.[35–38]
- Having more bulk in certain areas can help preventing orocutaneous fistulae.
- An ALT can be harvested simultaneously with a 2-team approach, while the resection is being done, without the need to postpone or to reposition the patient.
- An ALT can safely supply at least 150 cm^2 based on a single perforator.[39]
- The donor site of an ALT can almost always be repaired without the need of a skin graft. Even when the defect is too wide to be closed directly, a local flap either on a random vascular supply or on a small perforator can be lifted and rotated to facilitate closure.

Standard Setup

The setup can obviously vary depending on circumstances and, more importantly, depending on the type of robotic devices the reconstructive team has available.

In general terms, this type of procedure ideally requires 2 experienced surgeons, one at the console, controlling the robotic arms, one at the patient's head directly operating with 2 long metal suckers (**Fig. 2**).

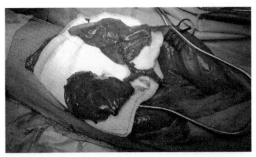

Fig. 1. Intraoperative picture of a chimeric Anterolateral Thigh Flap. 2 separate sets of blood vessels are feeding skin paddle and vastus lateralis compound.

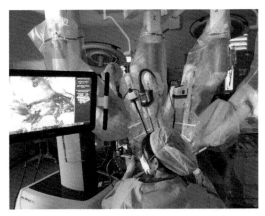

Fig. 2. Intraoperative set up of Da Vinci robotic system (Intuitive Inc, Sunnyvale CA). Transoral positioning of robotic arms and suctioning cannulas.

The role of the former being obvious, the role of the latter is quite essential too.

A radical difference between TORS and abdominal robotic surgery is that the operating field is not inflatable, or expansible.

There is room for only 2 robotic arms (1 with a forceps and 1 with a needle holder) and the main operator have to constantly rely on an assistant to create and maintain room for the optics by pushing and holding tissue while we inset the flap (**Fig. 3**).

This is especially important at the beginning when the free flap has very few if not none points of anchoring.

The operator at the patient's side also needs to assist suctioning blood and secretions and help maintaining the optics clean (**Fig. 4**).

Although it is known as an assistance role, the skills required are not trivial. The surgeon in that

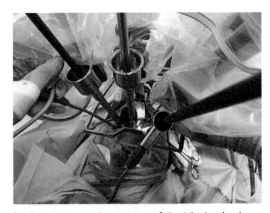

Fig. 3. Intraoperative set up of Da Vinci robotic system (Intuitive Inc, Sunnyvale CA). Surgeon at the patient's side assisting with retraction and suction while using the robot for insetting the free flap.

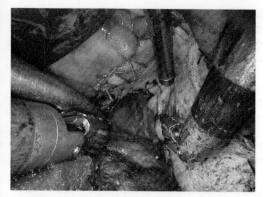

Fig. 4. Intraoperative image of a free flap being inset for an Oropharyngeal reconstruction. 2 robotic arms and 2 metal suctioning cannulas are visible.

position needs to be familiar with the procedure and anticipate needs and requirements and needs to be able to operate instrument without direct view of the field, but rather through a video visual feedback in a laparoscopic fashion we might say.

Setting up the robotic arms transorally can be a challenge as the space is tight and each arm needs some room to move avoiding clashing.

2 types of self-retractor are generally used, either an FK-WO TORS retractor (Olympus) or a standard Davis Boyle retractor for tonsillectomy which has less regulations and adjustments than the FK but takes out less space.

Given the metal instrumentation and the considerable force exerted, something like a Bite Raising Appliance is recommended to avoid dental damage during the procedure.

Refinements

Perforator location

Once a perforator has been identified, it is important to visualize how the flap is going to fit into the defect and design the flap in a way that positions the perforator in a well-protected area.

For example, reconstructing a lateral pharynx and soft palate defect, the area that reconstruct the soft palate is naturally going to have skin facing the oral cavity and fascial tissue facing the nasal cavity, left for secondary healing.

Having the perforator piercing the fascia in an area exposed to nasal secretions may pose a risk for the survival of the flap.

Making sure that the design of the skin paddle maintains the perforator safely protected within the parapharyngeal space can save some complications later.

Perfusion imaging

ALT angiosome has been widely investigated[32,40] and proven to have a reliable perfusion even for wide skin paddles[39] and an eccentric perforator can easily safely supply more distant and peripheral areas.

Oropharyngeal reconstruction, for anatomic reasons, needs to be truly 3 dimensional with often complex shapes with folding and partial rotation of portion of the flap.

The tissue transferred after tumor ablation provides cover for major blood vessels and cranial nerves, separates oral cavity secretions from the neck, provides bulk for the tongue base and pliability for the oral tongue and the palate.

Due to the complexity it is possible to incur in the occasional peripheral partial loss or even just a small dehiscence.

And even a small dehiscence or partial loss, in some cases, can cause severe complications.

In recent years Indocyanine Green has gained popularity as a rather simple technique to assess vascular perfusion of a given anatomic area.

There are several studies confirming both the feasibility and the benefits of this technique[41,42] and certainly it is something that should be taken into account in the context of complex head and neck reconstruction such as robotically inset perforator free flaps, especially considered the fact that even the smallest amount of peripheral loss or dehiscence, would be extremely difficult to repair without the use of the robot and therefore another general anesthetic.

A relatively quick intraoperative assessment could save some complications later.

Barb thread sutures

In setting the flap in the lowest part of the pharynx, even with the help of a robot, remains challenging and, although the more experience we gain the more we learn to use visual feedback, the lack of haptic remains debilitating. Tying knots with surgical sutures can become a substantially lengthier process.

To try and reduce the overall operating time some surgeons use barb thread sutures (**Fig. 5**), at least in some areas of the inset, resulting in

- Less knots to tie
- The thread remains under tension during the inset and helps keeping the flap in position until all the stitching is done.

J shape needle

For those areas where single stitches are more appropriate, such as corners or cardinal points, it can be useful to use J shaped needles (**Fig. 6**) with a round body.

While the round body helps not to cut through mucosa considering that the robot can exert considerably more force than what we perceive,

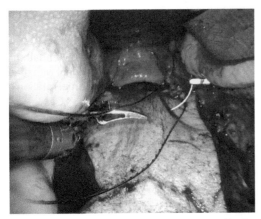

Fig. 5. Detail of barb thread surgical suture for free flap inset.

the J shape helps to grasp a deeper bite of tissue resulting in a more robust anchoring.

It is important not to forget that bigger flaps for complex cases have a bigger mass and, being inset vertically along the pharyngeal wall, are constantly under gravity pull. A deep and more robust anchoring point on prevertebral fascia can be extremely helpful to avoid sagging.

Another way to support a bulky flap against gravity and, at the same time add a more robust anchor point is a trans cervical stitch placed with a combination of transoral and tran cervical manouvers and ultimately looping around the hyoid bone.

Robot Assisted Microvascular Anastomosis

Further development of RAFFI reconstruction has naturally led to robotic assisted microvascular

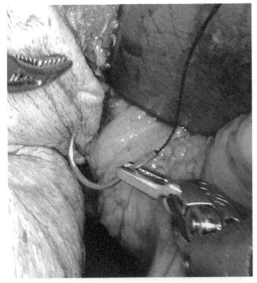

Fig. 6. Detail of J shaped needle for free flap inset.

anastomosis which has been documented to be both feasible and safe, although not superior and often more time consuming than hand sewn anastomosis.[43]

More robotic devices are becoming available, some like the Symani surgical system (Medical Microinstruments, Calci, Italy) are designed and engineered specifically for microsurgery.[44]

The aim is to be able, with the help of machines, to perform equally safe microvascular anastomosis on smaller vessels and in deeper recesses.

Once an established practice, this will allow surgeons to use perforator flaps with very short pedicles, even perforator to perforator type of anastomosis and to continue to progress on the pathway of minimising morbidity for the patients both functionally and cosmetically.

Limitations

Caution needs to be used as not all cases are suitable for TORS.

It is fair to say that robotic instrumentation is not always needed to inset flaps even after TORS[45] and not the whole flap needs to be inset robotically. It is often possible to do at least some of the inset transorally under direct vision and that can be helpful especially for the first few stitches to tack the flap on the main cardinal points. Thus, reducing the burden and the visual obstacle while handling a large skin paddle through the robot only.

Trismus is a major factor, together with the patient mandibular anatomy. Class II occlusions are associated with reduced oropharyngeal space[46] and reduced mouth opening.

A reassessment with examination under anesthesia to evaluate the feasibility of a TORS approach remains fundamental.

Although some authors describe reduced operating time compared to open surgery[19] the vast majority show a substantially longer time for TORS procedures,[4] with a systematic review calculating an average operating time of 710 minutes.[47]

The shorter operating time reports might account for small primary resections while the real challenge remain recurrence cases, for which the total operating time still remain high.

Nevertheless, it is important to appreciate the reduction in long term morbidity such as reducing risk of ORN and minimising scars.

Short term complications have to be looked carefully.

It may be true that robotic cases show lower postoperative complications but needs to be said that cases not suitable for TORS, therefore

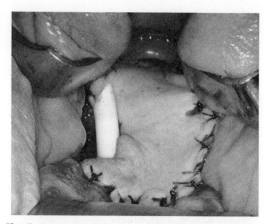

Fig. 7. Intraoperative view of free flap inset extending from soft palate to lateral pharynx and hypopharynx, down to the level of the epiglottis.

ending with an open surgery, are by definition more advanced, often with invasion of bone and extrinsic muscles.

Discussion

Perforator free flaps have allowed surgeons to reconstruct bigger defects, in a more tailored fashion and with reduced morbidity for the donor sites.

Transoral robotic reconstruction has allowed to reduce morbidity for the patients both from a functional point of view as well as cosmetic.

A systematic review from August 2023 identified a total of 132 patients having had robotic free flap reconstruction following HNC ablation. It showed an average length of stay of 13.5 days and a low rate for serious complications.[47]

Another literature review from October 2023 documented 100% flap survival[48] overall confirming it to be a safe procedure with low morbidity, despite

remaining, looking at published volume of cases, a niche procedure.

Having said that, the indications for RAFFI inset sit in a rather specific/small window.

It is between cases that can be operated with TORS but do not need free flap reconstruction and cases where because of trismus or invasion TORS is not possible and an open surgery is required.

It is mostly patients relapsing after previous treatments but still caught in time before cancer invades bone and masticatory muscles.

In the instance a trans robotic approach can provide reduced long-term morbidity with acceptable oncological outcomes, Given the above, RAFFI should not be regarded as a new default approach to all oropharyngeal recurrent tumors, much rather as new additional treatment option or a new surgical tool available for the reconstructive surgeon.

With correct indications and in the hands of an experienced team RAFFI can support in reconstructing big and complex defects covering areas (Fig. intraop) extending from soft palate to the level of the epiglottis (**Figs. 7** and **8**).

It is important that the reconstructive team embarking on robotic free flap reconstruction are not just familiar but comfortable with standard open approaches.

It is not simply because it may become necessary to convert from transoral to open, but also because a sound experience in traditional open surgery is fundamental to master the intricacies generated by trying to achieve the same primary objectives of a traditional approach but through a much smaller access and by proxy of a robotic device

It is important to be confident in both robotic surgery and free tissue transfer surgery and, since RAFFI is not an ideal technique for all cases, it is fundamental to have the necessary knowledge

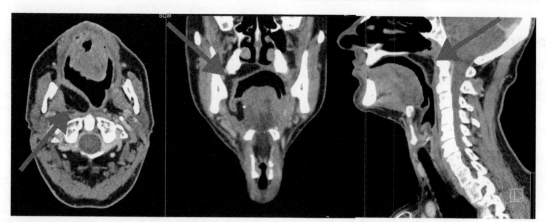

Fig. 8. Postoperative computed tomography scan showing the size and anatomic extension of the robotically inset free flap.

and experience to evaluate and assess each case, balancing out indications and contraindications: to understand which patients will benefit from it and which will not.

There are devices like the Da Vinci Single Port which has a single arm, rather than 3, which splits and opens up once on target leaving more space for maneuvering in the oral cavity.

Progressive refinements of robotic devices will bring smaller and less bulky instruments which will facilitate the work of the surgeon.

SUMMARY

Both perforator flaps and robotic surgery have at their core the concept of minimizing morbidity compared to traditional techniques.

Provided exclusion criteria are kept in consideration, robotic assisted perforator flaps inset can provide reconstruction for challenging recurrent oropharyngeal cancer cases, reducing the morbidity of surgical access, sparing important structures for swallow and speech function and reducing the impact of visible scars.

Future developments will benefit from the continuous refinements of technology in this field.

CLINICS CARE POINTS

- Refinements in stitching techniques for robotic inset.
- Inset technique combining robotic and hand sewn stitches.
- Use of Indocyanine green for perfusion study of perforator flap.
- Importance of respecting indications for robotic cases.

DISCLOSURE

The authors have no financial interest related to matters or materials discussed in this article to disclose.

REFERENCES

1. Alice Q L, Thomas D M. Decisional regret, symptom burden, and quality of life following transoral robotic surgery for oropharyngeal cancer Jamie Jae Young Kwon. Eitan Prisman. Oral Oncology 2023;146: 106537.
2. Matt Lechner, Liu Jacklyn, Masterson Liam, et al. HPV-associated oropharyngeal cancer: epidemiology, molecular biology and clinical management. Nat Rev Clin Oncol 2022;19(5):306–27.
3. Verduijn a Gerda M, Nienke D Sijtsema, Yvette van Norden, et al. Accounting for fractionation and heterogeneous dose distributions in the modelling of osteoradionecrosis in oropharyngeal carcinoma treatment. Radiother Oncol 2023;188:109889.
4. Liu H, Wang Y, Wu C, et al. Robotic compared with open operations for cancers of the head and neck: a systematic review and meta-analysis. Brit J Oral Max Fan Surg 2019;57(10):967–76.
5. Ang KK, Harris J, Wheeler R, et al. Human papillomavirus and survival of patients with oropharyngeal cancer. N Engl J Med 2010;363:24–35. https://doi.org/10.1056/NEJMoa0912217.
6. Zimmermann PH, Marijn S, Nora W, et al. Upfront Surgery vs. Primary Chemoradiation in an Unselected, Bicentric Patient Cohort with Oropharyngeal Squamous Cell Carcinoma—A Matched-Pair Analysis. Cancers (Basel) 2021;13(21):5265.
7. Theresa G, Stephen Y K, Ezra E WC. Current perspectives on recurrent HPV-mediated oropharyngeal cancer. Front Oncol 2022. https://doi.org/10.3389/fonc.2022.966899.
8. Hamoir M, Schmitz S, Suarez C, et al. The current role of salvage surgery in recurrent head and neck squamous cell carcinoma. Cancers 2018;10:E267. https://doi.org/10.3390/cancers10080267.
9. Wolf GT, Fisher SG. Induction chemo plus radiation compared with surgery plus radiation in patients with advanced laryngeal cancer. N Engl Med 1991;324:1685–90.
10. Campbell BH, Spinelli K. Aspiration Weight loss and quality of life in head and neck cancer survivors. Arch Otolaryngol Head Neck Surg 2004;130:1100–3.
11. O'Malley Jr BW, Weinstein GS, Snyder W, et al. Transoral robotic surgery(TORS) for base of tongue neoplasms. Laryngoscope 2006;116:1465–72.
12. Weinstein GS, Malley, Snyder W, et al. Transoral roboticsurgery: radical tonsillectomy. Arch Otolaryngol Head Neck Surg 2007;133:1220–6.
13. Moore EJ, Olsen KD, Kasperbauer JL. Transoral robotic surgery fororopharyngeal squamous cell carcinoma: a prospective study of feasibil-ity and functional outcomes. Laryngoscope 2009;119:2156–64.
14. Weinstein GS, O'Malley Jr BW, Cohen MA, et al. Transoral roboticsurgery for advanced oropharyngeal carcinoma. Arch Otolaryngol Head Neck Surg 2010;136:1079–85.
15. Jesse CS. Transoral robotic reconstruction of oropharyngeal defects: a case series. Plast Reconstr Surg 2010 Dec;126(6):1978–87.
16. Mehanna H, Kong A, Ahmed S. Recurrent head and neck cancer: United Kingdom National Multidisciplinary Guidelines. J Laryngol Otol 2016;130:S181–90. https://doi.org/10.1017/S002221511600061X.

17. Paleri V, Fox H, Coward S, et al. Transoral robotic surgery for residual and recurrent oropharyngeal cancers: exploratory study of surgical innovation using the IDEAL framework for early-phase surgical studies. Head Neck 2018;40:512–25. https://doi.org/10.1002/hed.25032.

18. Hilliary W, Samuel F, Benjamin B, et al. Salvage Surgery for Recurrent Cancers of the Oropharynx: comparing TORS With Standard Open Surgical Approaches. JAMA Otolaryngol Head Neck Surg 2013;139(8):773–8. https://doi.org/10.1001/jamaoto.2013.3866.

19. David Vir P, Constanza Viña S, Jordi VP, et al. Oropharyngeal free flap reconstruction: Transoral robotic surgery versus open approach. Laryngoscope Investigative Otolaryngology 2023;8:1564–70.

20. White H, Ford S, Bush B, et al. Salvage surgery for recurrent cancers of the oropharynx: comparing TORS with standard open surgical approaches. JAMA Otolaryngol Head Neck Surg 2013;139(8):773–8. https://doi.org/10.1001/jamaoto.2013.3866.

21. Young Min P, Hyung Kwon B, Hyun Pil C, et al. Comparison study of transoral robotic surgery and radical open surgery for hypopharyngeal cancer. Acta Otolaryngol 2013;133:641–8.

22. Chloe S, George G, Konstantinos C, et al. The perception of scar cosmesis following thyroid and parathyroid surgery: A prospective cohort study Asit Arora. Int J Surg 2016;25:38–43.

23. Song HG, Yun IS, Lee WJ, et al. Robot-assisted free flap in head and neck reconstruction. Arch Plast Surg 2013;40:353–8.

24. Almeida de JR, Park RC, Villanueva NL, et al. Reconstructive algorithm and classification system for transoral oropharyngeal defects. Head Neck 2014;36:934–41.

25. de Almeida JR, Park RC, Genden EM. Reconstruction of transoral robotic surgery defects: principles and techniques. J Reconstr Microsurg 2012;28:465–72.

26. Head and neck reconstruction. Neligan PC, Gullane P. In: Blondeel PN, Morris SF, Hallock GG, et al, editors. Perforator flaps: anatomy, technique and clinical applica- tions. St. Louis, MO: Quality Medical Publishing; 2006. p. 758–74.

27. Koshima I, Soeda S. Inferior epigastric artery skin flaps without rectus abdominis muscle. Br J Plast Surg 1989;42:645–8.

28. Song YG, Chen GZ, Song YL. The free thigh flap: a new free flap concept based on the septocutaneous artery. Br J Plast Surg 1984;37(2):149–59.

29. Koshima I, Yamamoto H, Hosoda M, et al. Free combined composite flaps using the lateral circumflex femoral system for repair of massive defects of the head and neck regions: an introduction to the chimeric flap principle. Plast Reconstr Surg 1993;92:411–20.

30. Koshima I, Fukuda H, Yamamoto H, et al. Free anterolateral thigh flaps for reconstruction of head and neck defects. Plast Reconstr Surg 1993;92:421–8.

31. Zaretski A, Wei FC, Lin CH, et al. Anterolateral thigh perforator flaps in head and neck reconstruction. Semin Plast Surg 2006;20(2):64–72.

32. Wei FC, Jain V, Celik N, et al. Have we found an ideal soft-tissue flap? An experience with 672 anterolateral thigh flaps. Plast Reconstr Surg 2002;109(7):2219–26. discussion 2227-30.

33. Jagdeep SC, Joy Odili. Perforator Flaps in Head and Neck Reconstruction. Semin Plast Surg 2010;24(3):237–54. https://doi.org/10.1055/s-0030-1263066.

34. Zaretski A, Wei FC, Lin CH, et al. Anterolateral Thigh Perforator Flaps in Head and Neck Reconstruction. Semin Plast Surg 2006;20(2):64–72. PMCID: PMC2884773.

35. Andreas K, Neil SS, Batista da Silva NP, et al. Step-by-step guide to ultrasound-based design of alt flaps by the microsurgeon - Basic and advanced applications and device settings. J Plast Reconstr Aesthetic Surg 2020;73(6):1081–90. Epub 2019 Dec 1.

36. Hong JP, Choi DH, Suh H, et al. A new plane of elevation: the superficial fascial plane for perforator flap elevation. J Reconstr Microsurg 2014;30:491–6.

37. Suh YC, Kim SH, Baek WY, et al. Super-thin ALT flap elevation using preoperative color doppler ultrasound planning: identification of horizontally running pathway at the deep adipofascial layers. J Plast Reconstr Aesthet Surg 2022;75(2):665–73. https://doi.org/10.1016/j.bjps.2021.09.051.

38. Visconti G, Bianchi A, Hayashi A, et al. Thin and superthin perforator flap elevation based on preoperative planning with ultrahighfrequency ultrasound. Arch Plast Surg 2020;47(4):365–70.

39. Saad N, Cromack D, Wang H, et al. Surface to Perforator Index: Assessing the Importance of the Number of Perforators in Successful Harvesting of the Anterolateral Thigh Flap. PRS Global Open 2022;10(11 Suppl):7.

40. Taylor GI, Corlett RJ, Dhar SC, et al. The anatomical (angiosome) and clinical territories of cutaneous perforating arteries: development of the concept and designing safe flaps. Plast Reconstr Surg 2011;127:1447–59.

41. Sunil C, Soumya K, Raghav M, et al. Role of Indocyanine Green Angiography in Free Flap Surgery: A Comparative Outcome Analysis of a Single-Center Large Series of 877 Consecutive Free Flaps. Indian J Plast Surg 2023;56(3):208–17.

42. Kuan-Cheng C, Chih-Hsun L, Hsu M, et al. Outcome analysis of free flap reconstruction for head and neck cancer with intraoperative indocyanine green angiography. Journal Plast Aest Recon Surg 2023;85:387–92.

43. Chih-Sheng L, Chen-Te L, Shih-An L, et al. Robot-assisted microvascular anastomosis in head and neck free flap reconstruction: Preliminary experiences and results. Microsurgery 2019;1–6. https://doi.org/10.1002/micr.30458.

44. Nicole L, Lisanne G, Anna W, et al. Early Experience Using a New Robotic Microsurgical System for Lymphatic Surgery. PRS Global Open 2022.

45. Hatten KM, Brody RM, Weinstein GS, et al. Defining the role of free flaps for transoral robotic surgery. Ann Plast Surg 2018;80:45–9.

46. Kim M, Hwang CJ, Cha JY, et al. Correlation Analysis between Three-Dimensional Changes in Pharyngeal Airway Space and Skeletal Changes in Patients with Skeletal Class II Malocclusion following Orthognathic Surgery. BioMed Res Int 2022;2022:3995690. PMID: 35059461; PMCID: PMC8766181.

47. Monroe D, Pyne JM, McLennan S, et al. Characteristics and outcomes of transoral robotic surgery with free-flap reconstruction for oropharyngeal cancer: a systematic review. J Robot Surg 2023;17(4):1287–97. Epub 2023 Mar 25. PMID: 36964850. It is probably safe to correlate the operating time with the complexity of the resection and therefore the reconstruction.

48. Rehman U, Whiteman E, Sarwar MS, et al. Reconstruction of head and neck oncological soft tissue defects post-resection using robotic surgery: a systematic review of the current literature. Br J Oral Maxillofac Surg 2023;61(8):514–21. Epub 2023 Aug 5. PMID: 37661537.

Current and Future Implications of Lymphedema Surgery in Head and Neck Reconstruction

Sonia Kukreja-Pandey, MD[a], Miguel Angel Gaxiola-Garcia, MD[b],
Nishan Moheeputh, MD[c], Wei F. Chen, MD[a],*

KEYWORDS

- Head and neck lymphedema • Face swelling • Head and neck cancer
- Lymphaticovenular anastomosis • Lymph node to vein anastomosis • Cervical lymph nodes
- Neurodegenerative disorders

KEY POINTS

- Despite significant strides in managing extremity lymphedema, head and neck lymphedema (HNL) has been overlooked.
- Internal swelling, affecting mucosal and submucosal tissues, is more prevalent in HNL compared to external swelling, involving the skin and subcutaneous layers.
- Traditional conservative modalities used for extremity lymphedema management, such as compression garments, pneumatic compression, and manual lymphatic drainage, are difficult to apply to the head and neck region.
- Lymphatic surgical procedures, notably lymphaticovenular anastomosis (LVA), lymph node-to-vein anastomosis (LNVA), and debulking liposuction have been attempted and show promising outcomes.
- Treatment of HNL may extend its effects intracranially, due to the interconnectedness of lymphatic systems.

INTRODUCTION

In the wake of significant advancements made in the treatment of extremity lymphedema over the last decade, attention has increasingly turned to the intricate and often overlooked head and neck regions. The impact of lymphedema on these areas, regardless of its etiology, manifests not just physically but also functionally, often eluding sufficient medical intervention.[1–4] Even though a significant proportion of head and neck cancer survivors are affected by lymphedema, the condition remains underdiagnosed due to its subtler presentation, particularly when it occurs without a clear initiating event.

The reality that such a critical condition has remained relatively in the shadows underscores the need for increased awareness and expertise in the diagnosis and treatment of head and neck lymphedema (HNL). Through dedicated research and clinical practice, there has been noteworthy advancement in the fundamental understanding and early surgical management of lymphedema,

[a] Department of Plastic and Reconstructive Surgery, Cleveland Clinic Foundation, 9500 Euclid Avenue, Cleveland, OH 44195, USA; [b] Hospital Infantil de México "Federico Gómez" (Mexico's Children's Hospital), Dr Marquez 162, 06720 Cuauhtemoc, Mexico City, Mexico; [c] Med Esthetique, 75 Royal Road, Petit Raffray, Mauritius 30711
* Corresponding author.
E-mail address: chenw6@ccf.org

Oral Maxillofacial Surg Clin N Am 36 (2024) 567–574
https://doi.org/10.1016/j.coms.2024.07.007

especially of the limbs. The commitment to this field over the last decade has set the stage for innovative developments in lymphatic reconstruction, aiming for not just management but reversal of the condition.[5,6]

As the researchers seek to bring these advancements to the forefront of HNL management, this article serves as a platform to share the accumulated knowledge and strategic approaches that have been effective in limb lymphedema. By doing so, the researchers contribute to a broader conversation on addressing a condition that, until recently, has not received the attention it deserves, with the goal of extending these successes to benefit those suffering from HNL.

ANATOMY

The gravity of HNL may not always be appreciable on inspection of the patient as fluid accumulates not only in the subcutaneous space (external) but also in the submucosal space (internal). Most patients with external edema present with periorbital, cheek, and/or submental neck swelling due to the superficial fat compartments corresponding to these regions.[7] The swelling distribution depends on the site and extent of lymphatic injury as well as the compensatory mechanisms like collateralization within the lymphatic system. A thorough understanding of the anatomy of head and neck lymphatic system is crucial for understanding the pathogenesis of the disease.[8] While cervical lymph nodes have been extensively studied, the lymphatic system anatomy cranial to the neck remains less elucidated.[9] In this regard, cadaver injection studies have provided valuable insights into the lymphatic vessels and nodes anatomy in the scalp and face.[10,11] For instance, frontal scalp and upper and lower eyelids drain into obliquely running lymph collectors across the medial cheek, ultimately reaching the buccinator lymph node and submandibular lymph nodes. Similarly, the frontotemporal scalp and eyelids drain into preauricular lymph nodes and parotid nodes. The temporoparietal and occipital scalp drain into retroauricular and occipital lymph nodes, respectively.[10,11]

The arrangement of lymphatic vessels in the head and neck differs from that found in the extremities. Notably, the lymphatic capillaries are present not only in the dermis but also in the galea, contrasting with solely dermal lymphatic capillaries seen elsewhere. Additionally, the lymphatic collectors that receive drainage from both dermis and galea are situated in a more superficial fat plane as compared to those in extremities (**Figs. 1** and **2**).[10,11] The lymphatic drainage within the mucosal linings of the head and neck is relatively less well understood.

The HNL system is not limited to the extracranial region. The brain also has a lymphatic system of its own, comprising glial cells lined perivascular space (glymphatics) and a network of lymphatics along the dural sinuses (meningeal lymphatics).[12–14] The cerebrospinal fluid flows in the periarterial spaces of brain parenchyma, mixes with the interstitial fluid, and exits through the perivenous space, sweeping away the brain's waste in the process.[13] The intermixed cerebrospinal fluid (CSF) and interstitial fluid constitute the brain lymph that drains into the dural venous sinuses (fluid) and into the meningeal lymphatics (macromolecules) lying along them. The meningeal lymphatics exit the skull predominantly through the orbit, nose (cribriform plate), and jugular foramen, ultimately draining into the deep cervical lymph nodes.[15–17]

DIAGNOSIS

Diagnosing HNL presents distinctive challenges that set it apart from its extremity counterpart. The detection and quantification of the "external" and "internal" swelling of the head and neck require additional tools to assist clinical examination.[18–22] In many cases, patients experience internal swelling without the external manifestations that typically herald lymphedema, making detection difficult.[3,23,24] Subtle indicators, such as mild or bilateral external swelling, particularly localized in the neck, or alterations due to surgical interventions, may obscure the true extent of the condition. The diurnal variation of symptoms—with worsening in the morning that improves as the day progresses—further complicates diagnosis during routine clinical hours. There is often a lack of recognition of internal lymphedema's "symptoms," emphasizing the need for thorough clinical assessments.

Existing clinical grading systems for HNL consider factors such as swelling reversibility, fibrotic development, and skin changes, paralleling those for extremity lymphedema.[4] For facial volume, standardized tape measurements based on anatomic landmarks facilitate the calculation of a "composite facial score" and a "composite neck score." However, the precise identification of these landmarks can be problematic in cases of significant lymphedema, marked obesity, or postsurgical anatomic changes.[25] The accuracy of these measurements is also susceptible to variables such as the patient's positioning, involuntary facial movements, and the applied tension on the measuring tape. Moreover, tape measurement is inherently subject to substantial variability between different observers and even with repeated measures by the same observer. Given these limitations, tape

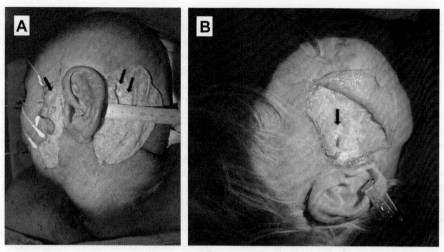

Fig. 1. (*A*) Exploration of preauricular and postauricular regions in a non-embalmed human cadaver. Two lymphatic collectors were observed in the postauricular region, superficial to the galea aponeurosis, located 2 to 3 cm posterior to the retroauricular groove. (*B*) Preauricular region showed one lymphatic collector in the subcutaneous layer, located about 2 cm anterior to the tip of the tragus.

measurements should be considered a supportive tool within a broader diagnostic framework rather than a definitive test. Its utility lies in its ability to provide additional data points that complement other diagnostic modalities, thereby enhancing the overall evaluation of HNL.

Bioimpedance spectroscopy has emerged as a promising objective method to assess the extracellular fluid component of HNL.[26] While it is a proven diagnostic modality in extremity lymphedema with known diagnostic parameters that have been extensively investigated, such conditions for HNL are not in place yet. We expect future studies to bring this technology into a more mature application in diagnosing HNL.

Detecting functional deficits due to internal mucosal and submucosal swelling is inherently more complex than identifying external swelling. Patients may exhibit a spectrum of oronasopharyngeal symptoms impacting swallowing, chewing, speech, and occasionally, breathing.[3] To assess these internal symptoms, evaluations often include speech and swallowing tests, while tools like the revised Patterson scale, administered through laryngoscopy examination, help quantify the internal swelling.[27] However, a primary limitation of this scale is its vulnerability to significant inter-rater variability. Additionally, its effectiveness depends on the clinician's experience, with less seasoned practitioners possibly struggling to assess the severity of swelling accurately.

Patient-reported symptom scores serve as reliable indicators for tracking the disease over time. Individuals with early-stage HNL may report feelings

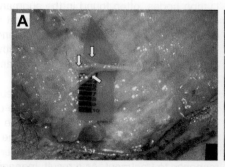
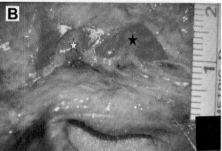

Fig. 2. (*A*) Exploration of preauricular region in another cadaver showed 3 lymphatic collectors in the subcutaneous plane, adherent to each other. The vessels were separated out superiorly to measure their external diameter, which ranged from 0.2 to 0.3 mm. (*B*) In the same cadaver, 2 lymph nodes were identified about 1.4 cm anterior to the tip of tragus. The superior lymph node (black star) was superficial to superficial musculoaponeurotic system (SMAS), while the inferior lymph node (white star) was deep to the SMAS.

of fullness or tension, despite the absence of visible swelling. Chronic conditions can present a diverse array of symptoms due to swelling, fibrosis, and consequent impairment of joint movement, paresthesia, and pain. The Head and Neck Lymphedema and Fibrosis Symptom Inventory rates a wide array of symptoms on a 5 point scale and has shown promise for monitoring patient outcomes.[28]

Currently, indocyanine green lymphography (ICGL) stands as the most dependable diagnostic technique for HNL. This protocol, adapted from the proven methodologies for extremity lymphedema, enables comprehensive mapping of the lymphatic territories in the facial, scalp, and neck regions. ICGL provides critical insights into lymphatic functionality and pathology, including fluorophore transit times, the layout of lymph collectors, and the presence of collateral or dermal backflow pathways. It also establishes a baseline for assessing treatment effectiveness through subsequent ICGL evaluations. While ICGL stands as the primary diagnostic tool, its efficacy is maximized when complemented by other diagnostic techniques mentioned earlier, tailored to the individual patient's unique presentation, thus ensuring an effective approach to HNL diagnosis.[29–32]

SURGICAL TREATMENT STRATEGIES

Similar to the approach in extremity lymphedema, conservative treatments are prioritized in managing HNL.[33] Manual lymph drainage (MLD) and compression therapy stand as the foundational nonsurgical interventions.[34–36] However, the efficacy of MLD can be compromised when patients are tasked with self-administration, leading to potential inconsistencies in technique and frequency. Moreover, adherence to using facial and neck compression garments is notably low, largely due to social stigma and discomfort associated with their use. Pneumatic compression devices have been introduced to enhance the effects of MLD, providing an option for home treatment. Despite this, their bulky nature and the discomfort they can cause often lead to patient dissatisfaction and decreased usage.[36–38]

While conservative treatments including MLD and compression therapy are essential in managing HNL, the transition to surgical options is often hesitated, even when the nonsurgical treatments had proven unsuccessful. This reluctance stems from the lymphedema surgeons' limited experience with HNL, the uncertainty regarding the success of surgical methods that are well established in extremity lymphedema, and the relatively benign natural progression of HNL, attributed to the anatomic advantages of the head and neck

region and gravitational drainage. Additionally significant consideration is the life expectancy of patients, particularly those with HNL secondary to cancer treatment, where the focus tends to prioritize life-extending treatments over lymphedema management.

For patients with severe HNL who do not respond to conservative treatments, surgical options become a viable treatment option. Techniques adapted from extremity lymphedema management, including debulking and physiologic surgeries, have demonstrated effectiveness in the head and neck region.[39–43] While existing literature often overlooks the impact on internal swelling, clinical experience suggests that successful external swelling reduction through these surgeries often correlates with significant improvement and regeneration in the regional lymphatic system, demonstrable through ICGL.[44] Consequently, it is reasonable to expect that the alleviation of external symptoms will be paralleled by internal improvements, as evidenced by postoperative assessments.

Lymphaticovenular anastomosis (LVA) and lymph node-to-vein anastomosis (LNVA) have proven effective for reducing swelling in the periorbital, cheek, and scalp areas. These procedures utilize diagnostic mapping techniques such as ultra-high frequency ultrasound, ICGL, isosulfan blue dye, and occasionally radioisotopes to identify optimal surgical sites.[45–48] The cheeks, preauricular region, postauricular scalp, and mandibular area are commonly chosen for LVA, with a preference for the preauricular region due to its favorable accessibility through a facelift preauricular incision.[49–53] The decision on the surgical site should be guided by the potential to access lymph vessels of the highest quality and least pathologic impact, as well as the surgeon's goal for the number of LVAs to perform. Fewer LVAs may be needed if the lymph vessels are of high quality. Lymph nodes, often found in the submandibular, preauricular, postauricular, and occipital regions, may vary due to previous ablative surgeries. Surgeons should adapt their approach to either LVA, LNVA, or both, based on the condition and availability of lymph vessels and nodes.[50,54]

Extrapolating from the experience in treating extremity lymphedema, it appears that the effect of gravity on the lymph drainage and the relative position of the affected region from the central lymphatic system affect disease severity and response to treatment. As a result, managing lymphedema in the arms is generally less complex compared to the thighs and legs, with the feet being notably more difficult to treat. The anatomic positioning of the head and neck, being higher and closer to the central lymphatic system, along with the positive effects of gravity, gives these areas an advantage in treatment effectiveness. LVA and LNVA procedures in the head and neck regions are expected to be more effective compared to their performance on other body parts.

Debulking surgeries, such as lower eyelid blepharoplasty for severe eyelid swelling and submental liposuction for anterior neck swelling, have shown benefits in enhancing both appearance and functional outcomes, such as improved vision and quality of life.[55–58] In a manner akin to the treatment of extremity lymphedema, these debulking procedures can be effectively paired with physiologic surgeries such as LVA and LNVA.[59] This combination leverages the regenerative capacity of the lymphatic system following the surgical removal of the pathologic tissue affected by lymphedema, optimizing the overall therapeutic outcome.[39]

In the realm of HNL treatment, other physiologic procedures including vascularized lymph node transfer (VLNT) and vascularized lymph vessel transfer (VLVT) remained undocumented. Free tissue transfers, a "robbing Peter to pay Paul" approach, necessitate significant lymphatic disruption at the donor site and are markedly more invasive than both LVA and LNVA. In the senior author (W.F.C.)'s opinion, VLNT, with its considerable donor site morbidity, is now considered more of historical interest. VLVT, though still a worthy consideration in the surgical armamentarium for lymphedema, should be reserved as a last option, contemplated only after LVA and LNVA have been exhausted.[40]

The effectiveness of HNL surgeries is evaluated using various measures, including the reduction of visible swelling, skin pinch thickness, changes in facial circumference, and patient-reported outcomes. Improvements can be observed as early as 4 days to 6 months post-surgery, according to literature.[50–52] In our practice, patients often perceive immediate benefits postoperatively, with continuous improvement over 1 to 2 years. Among the various methods for tracking surgical outcomes, ICGL and patient-reported outcomes are particularly valuable. They offer a detailed and specific assessment of the patient's response to the surgical intervention, capturing both the immediate success of the procedure and the long-term progress.

FUTURE DIRECTIONS

The detrimental impact of HNL is undeniable, particularly the impairment of vital functions like eating and speaking, thereby diminishing the quality of life. The current landscape of HNL management reveals that, unlike extremity lymphedema, compression garments play a limited role, and reliance on MLD, whether self-administered or therapist-led, is insufficient. Surgical interventions for HNL, however, hold the promise of arresting disease progression and enhancing patient well-being. To accurately evaluate treatment efficacy, there is a pressing need to refine and standardize outcome measures, incorporating tools like ICGL and patient-reported outcomes to garner robust data.

LVA and LNVA procedures especially in primary lymphedema consistently show that their therapeutic benefits extend beyond the immediate area of surgical intervention, alleviating regional (limb) swelling, and also diminishing systemic swelling. Patients with primary lymphedema affecting both the face and limbs have reported significant facial swelling reduction, corresponding with limb swelling decrease, after undergoing limb surgery. This symptom relief frequently extends to mucosal areas including the gums, nasal passages, and pharynx, highlighting the widespread regional and systemic benefits of such surgeries. These outcomes suggest that effective treatment can be achieved even when the surgery is performed away from the direct site of the problem. The capacity for successful surgical outcomes in distant anatomic regions reinforces the concept that lymphatic reconstruction need not be localized to exert its effects. Additionally, reports of enhanced cognitive functions postsurgery, such as improved critical thinking and memory, alongside the lifting of "brain fog," have led to the hypothesis of a connection between extracranial lymphatic reconstruction and intracranial fluid dynamics.

The evolving comprehension of the brain's lymphatic system, particularly its drainage into cervical nodes, underlines the potential impact of cervical lymph node removal, extending beyond the manifestations of external and internal lymphedema. The brain's lymphatic network, essential for eliminating waste and immune monitoring, is key in averting protein build-up linked to neurodegenerative disorders.[60–63] The intricate connection between the brain's internal lymphatic framework and the external cervical lymphatic system leads to the speculation that patients with HNL could face a heightened risk of cognitive impairments, highlighting the need for thorough cognitive function assessments following extensive neck surgeries, beyond the potential cognitive effects of chemotherapy.

Furthermore, this insight gives rise to another hypothesis that addressing HNL could either prevent or ameliorate cognitive deficits tied to lymphatic dysfunction in the head and neck area.[62,64] Observations of significant cognitive enhancement in Alzheimer's patients post-neck LVA support the notion that extracranial LVA might relieve brain lymphedema.[65,66] This idea emphasizes the dual advantages of lymphatic surgery for patients with HNL: reducing lymphedema symptoms and mitigating cognitive decline.

These hypotheses regarding brain lymphatics have already garnered international research interest, propelling further studies to deepen our grasp of the subject. The current endeavors in reconstructing HNL are paving the way for future explorations into brain lymphatic surgery.

CLINICS CARE POINTS

- As internal swelling is more common than external swelling in the HNL history and examination should include assessment of chewing, swallowing, speech, and breathing.

- Clinical examination should be supplemented with quality-of-life scores, face pictures, bioimpedance spectroscopy, ICGL, and laryngoscopy for accurate diagnosis and disease monitoring.

- Traditional conservative modalities used for extremity lymphedema management, such as compression garments, pneumatic compression, and manual lymphatic drainage, are difficult to apply to the head and neck region, hence the need to explore surgical options.

- Lymphatic surgical techniques used for extremity lymphedema, both physiologic and debulking procedures, have been anecdotally utilized in the head and neck with encouraging results.

- A better understanding of the HNL anatomy is being gained using ICG lymphography of patients with HNL and through cadaver dissections. The connectivity of the intracranial lymphatic system and the extracranial lymphatic system has been established suggesting that treatment of HNL may extend its effects intracranially.

DISCLOSURE

None of the authors has any conflicts of interest or financial interest in any of the products, devices, or drugs mentioned in this study. The study was not financially supported by any grants.

REFERENCES

1. Deng J, Ridner SH, Dietrich MS, et al. Prevalence of secondary lymphedema in patients with head and neck cancer. J Pain Symptom Manag 2012;43(2):244–52.

2. Jeans C, Brown B, Ward EC, et al. Comparing the prevalence, location, and severity of head and neck lymphedema after postoperative radiotherapy for oral cavity cancers and definitive chemoradiotherapy for oropharyngeal, laryngeal, and hypopharyngeal cancers. Head Neck 2020;42(11): 3364–74.

3. Jackson LK, Ridner SH, Deng J, et al. Internal Lymphedema Correlates with Subjective and Objective Measures of Dysphagia in Head and Neck Cancer Patients. J Palliat Med 2016;19(9):949–56.

4. Smith BG, Lewin JS. Lymphedema management in head and neck cancer. Curr Opin Otolaryngol Head Neck Surg 2010;18(3):153–8.

5. Chen WF, Ku YC, Yamamoto T, et al. Is Lymphedema Cure a Clinical Reality? Arch Plast Surg 2023;50(06): 635–6.

6. Scomacao I, Lensing JN, Bowen MJ, et al. Cure for Lymphedema: Myth or Reality. Plast Reconstr Surg Glob Open 2020;8(9 Suppl):72.

7. Schenck TL, Koban KC, Schlattau A, et al. The Functional Anatomy of the Superficial Fat Compartments of the Face: A Detailed Imaging Study. Plast Reconstr Surg 2018;141(6):1351–9.

8. Iwanaga J, Lofton C, He P, et al. Lymphatic System of the Head and Neck. J Craniofac Surg 2021;32(5): 1901–5.

9. Robbins KT, Clayman G, Levine PA, Medina J, Sessions R. Neck Dissection Classification Update Revisions Proposed by the American Head and Neck Society and the American Academy of Otolaryngology-Head and Neck Surgery.

10. Pan WR, Suami H, Taylor GI. Lymphatic drainage of the superficial tissues of the head and neck: Anatomical study and clinical implications. Plast Reconstr Surg 2008;121(5):1614–24.

11. Pan WR, Le Roux CM, Briggs CA. Variations in the lymphatic drainage pattern of the head and neck: Further anatomic studies and clinical implications. Plast Reconstr Surg 2011;127(2):611–20.

12. Louveau A, Harris TH, Kipnis J. Revisiting the Mechanisms of CNS Immune Privilege. Trends Immunol 2015;36(10):569–77.

13. Bohr T, Hjorth PG, Holst SC, et al. The glymphatic system: Current understanding and modeling. iScience 2022;25(9):1–33.

14. Aspelund A, Antila S, Proulx ST, et al. A dural lymphatic vascular system that drains brain interstitial fluid and macromolecules. J Exp Med 2015; 212(7):991–9.

15. Maloveska M, Danko J, Petrovova E, et al. Dynamics of Evans blue clearance from cerebrospinal fluid into

meningeal lymphatic vessels and deep cervical lymph nodes. Neurol Res 2018;40(5):372–80.

16. Albayram MS, Smith G, Tufan F, et al. Non-invasive MR imaging of human brain lymphatic networks with connections to cervical lymph nodes. Nat Commun 2022;13(1):1–14.

17. Xue Y, Liu X, Koundal S, et al. In vivo T1 mapping for quantifying glymphatic system transport and cervical lymph node drainage. Sci Rep 2020;10(1):1–13.

18. Arends CR, Lindhout JE, van der Molen L, et al. A systematic review of validated assessments methods for head and neck lymphedema. Eur Arch Oto-Rhino-Laryngol 2023;280(6):2653–61.

19. Spinelli BA. Head and Neck Lymphedema Assessment Methods. Rehabilitation Oncology 2021;39(4): E122–4.

20. Fadhil M, Singh R, Havas T, et al. Systematic review of head and neck lymphedema assessment. Head Neck 2022;44(10):2301–15.

21. Deng J, Ridner SH, Aulino JM, et al. Assessment and measurement of head and neck lymphedema state-of-the-science and future directions. Oral Oncol 2015;51(5):431–7.

22. Starmer H, Cherry MG, Patterson J, et al. Assessment of Measures of Head and Neck Lymphedema Following Head and Neck Cancer Treatment: A Systematic Review. Lymphatic Res Biol 2023;21(1): 42–51.

23. Deng J, Murphy BA, Dietrich MS, et al. Impact of secondary lymphedema after head and neck cancer treatment on symptoms, functional status, and quality of life. Head Neck 2013;35(7):1026–35.

24. Queija D dos S, Dedivitis RA, Arakawa-Sugueno L, et al. Cervicofacial and Pharyngolaryngeal Lymphedema and Deglutition After Head and Neck Cancer Treatment. Dysphagia 2020;35(3):479–91.

25. Chotipanich A, Kongpit N. Precision and reliability of tape measurements in the assessment of head and neck lymphedema. PLoS One 2020;15(5). https://doi.org/10.1371/JOURNAL.PONE.0233395.

26. Purcell A, Nixon J, Fleming J, et al. Measuring head and neck lymphedema: The "ALOHA" trial. Head Neck 2016;38(1):79–84.

27. Starmer HM, Drinnan M, Bhabra M, et al. Development and reliability of the revised Patterson Edema Scale. Clin Otolaryngol 2021;46(4):752–7.

28. Deng J, Murphy BA, Niermann KJ, et al. Validity Testing of the Head and Neck Lymphedema and Fibrosis Symptom Inventory. Lymphatic Res Biol 2022;20(6):629–39.

29. Amanda P, Andrew M, Hiroo S, et al. Lymphatic drainage patterns in head and neck lymphoedema: A preliminary imaging study with indocyanine green lymphography - Wounds International. Journal of Lymphedema 2023. Available at: https://wounds international.com/journal-articles/lymphatic-drain age-patterns-in-head-and-neck-lymphoedema-a-

preliminary-imaging-study-with-indocyanine-green-lymphography/. [Accessed 10 March 2024].

30. Narushima M, Yamamoto T, Ogata F, et al. Indocyanine Green Lymphography Findings in Limb Lymphedema. J Reconstr Microsurg 2016;32(1):72–9.

31. Yamamoto T, Iida T, Matsuda N, et al. Indocyanine green (ICG)-enhanced lymphography for evaluation of facial lymphoedema. J Plast Reconstr Aesthetic Surg 2011;64(11):1541–4.

32. Unno N, Nishiyama M, Suzuki M, et al. Quantitative Lymph Imaging for Assessment of Lymph Function using Indocyanine Green Fluorescence Lymphography. Eur J Vasc Endovasc Surg 2008;36(2):230–6.

33. Tyker A, Franco J, Massa ST, et al. Treatment for lymphedema following head and neck cancer therapy: A systematic review. Am J Otolaryngol 2019;40(5): 761–9.

34. Pigott A, Nixon J, Fleming J, et al. Head and neck lymphedema management: Evaluation of a therapy program. Head Neck 2018;40(6):1131–7.

35. Yao T, Beadle B, Holsinger CF, et al. Effectiveness of a Home-based Head and Neck Lymphedema Management Program: A Pilot Study. Laryngoscope 2020;130(12):E858–62.

36. Mayrovitz HN, Ryan S, Hartman JM. Usability of advanced pneumatic compression to treat cancer-related head and neck lymphedema: A feasibility study. Head Neck 2018;40(1):137–43.

37. Ridner SH, Dietrich MS, Deng J, et al. Advanced pneumatic compression for treatment of lymphedema of the head and neck: a randomized wait-list controlled trial. Support Care Cancer 2021;29(2): 795–803.

38. Gutierrez C, Karni RJ, Naqvi S, et al. Head and Neck Lymphedema: Treatment Response to Single and Multiple Sessions of Advanced Pneumatic Compression Therapy. Otolaryngol Head Neck Surg 2019; 160(4):622–6. Research Support, N.I.H., Extramural, Research Support, Non-U.S. Gov't.

39. Chen WF, Pandey SK, Lensing JN. Does Liposuction for Lymphedema Worsen Lymphatic Injury? Lymphology 2023;56(1):3–12.

40. Pandey SK, Fahradyan V, Orfahli LM, et al. Plastic and Aesthetic Research Supermicrosurgical lymphaticovenular anastomosis vs. vascularized lymph vessel transplant-technical optimization and when to perform which. Plast Aesthet Res 2021;8:47.

41. Schaverien MV, Badash I, Patel KM, et al. Vascularized Lymph Node Transfer for Lymphedema. Semin Plast Surg 2018;32(1):28–35.

42. Cakmakoglu C, Kwiecien GJ, Schwarz GS, et al. Lymphaticovenous Bypass for Immediate Lymphatic Reconstruction in Locoregional Advanced Melanoma Patients. J Reconstr Microsurg 2020;36(4): 247–52.

43. Chen WF. How to Get Started Performing Supermicrosurgical Lymphaticovenous Anastomosis to Treat

Lymphedema. Ann Plast Surg 2018;81(6S Suppl 1): S15–20.

44. Chen WF, Zhao H, Yamamoto T, et al. Indocyanine Green Lymphographic Evidence of Surgical Efficacy Following Microsurgical and Supermicrosurgical Lymphedema Reconstructions. J Reconstr Microsurg 2016;32(9):688–98.

45. Bourgeois P, Peters E, Van Mieghem A, et al. Edemas of the face and lymphoscintigraphic examination. Sci Rep 2021;11(1). https://doi.org/10.1038/s41598-021-85835-w.

46. Hara H, Mihara M. Multilymphosome injection indocyanine green lymphography can detect more lymphatic vessels than lymphoscintigraphy in lymphedematous limbs. J Plast Reconstr Aesthetic Surg 2020;73(6): 1025–30.

47. Chen WF, Pandey SK. Distal- to- proximal sequential ICG injection technique (DOPSIT) for lymphatic vessels mapping. Plast Aesthet Res 2023;10(1):null.

48. Hayashi A, Giacalone G, Yamamoto T, et al. Ultra High-frequency Ultrasonographic Imaging with 70 MHz Scanner for Visualization of the Lymphatic Vessels. Plast Reconstr Surg Glob Open 2019;7(1): e2086.

49. Mihara M, Uchida G, Hara H, et al. Lymphaticovenous anastomosis for facial lymphoedema after multiple courses of therapy for head-and-neck cancer. J Plast Reconstr Aesthetic Surg 2011;64(9):1221–5.

50. Koshima I, Imai H, Yoshida S, et al. Lymphaticovenular Anastomosis for Persistent Immunosuppressant-Related Eyelid Edema. International Microsurgery Journal 2018;2(2). https://doi.org/10.24983/scitemed. imj.2018.00090.

51. Inatomi Y, Yoshida S, Kamizono K, et al. Successful treatment of severe facial lymphedema by lymphovenous anastomosis. Head Neck 2018;40(7):E73–6.

52. Ayestaray B, Bekara F, Andreoletti JB. π-shaped lymphaticovenular anastomosis for head and neck lymphoedema: a preliminary study. J Plast Reconstr Aesthetic Surg 2013;66(2):201–6.

53. Ren ZH, Gu SL, Ji T, et al. Lymphatic-venous anastomosis for head and neck lymphedema using supermicrosurgery: case report and literature review. China J Oral Maxillofac Surg 2023;3:306–8.

54. Pak CS, Suh HP, Kwon JG, et al. Lymph Node to Vein Anastomosis (LNVA) for lower extremity lymphedema. J Plast Reconstr Aesthetic Surg 2021;74(9): 2059–67.

55. Sagili S, Selva D, Malhotra R. Eyelid lymphedema following neck dissection and radiotherapy. Ophthalmic Plast Reconstr Surg 2013;29(6). https://doi.org/10.1097/IOP.0B013E3182831C11.

56. Silverman AT, Hoffman R, Cohen M, et al. Severe cheek and lower eyelid lymphedema after resection of oropharyngeal tumor and radiation. J Craniofac Surg 2010;21(2):598–601.

57. Brake MK, Jain L, Hart RD, et al. Liposuction for submental lymphedema improves appearance and self-perception in the head and neck cancer patient. Otolaryngol Head Neck Surg 2014;151(2):221–5.

58. Alamoudi U, Taylor B, MacKay C, et al. Submental liposuction for the management of lymphedema following head and neck cancer treatment: a randomized controlled trial. Journal of Otolaryngology - Head & Neck Surgery 2018;47(1):22.

59. Chen WF. Is it Possible to Perform Lymphaticovenular Anastomosis after Liposuction for Lymphedema? J Chir 2016;12(4). https://doi.org/10.7438/1584-9341-12-4-7.

60. Cheng Y, Wang YJ. Meningeal Lymphatic Vessels: A Drain of the Brain Involved in Neurodegeneration? Neurosci Bull 2020;36(5):557–60.

61. Gallina P, Nicoletti C, Scollato A, et al. The "Glymphatic-Lymphatic System Pathology" and a New Categorization of Neurodegenerative Disorders. Front Neurosci 2021;15(May):1–3.

62. Hsu SJ, Zhang C, Jeong J, et al. Enhanced Meningeal Lymphatic Drainage Ameliorates Neuroinflammation and Hepatic Encephalopathy in Cirrhotic Rats. Gastroenterology 2021;160(4):1315–29.e13.

63. Zou W, Pu T, Feng W, et al. Blocking meningeal lymphatic drainage aggravates Parkinson's disease-like pathology in mice overexpressing mutated α-synuclein. Transl Neurodegener 2019;8(1):1–17.

64. Ding XB, Wang XX, Xia DH, et al. Impaired meningeal lymphatic drainage in patients with idiopathic Parkinson's disease. Nat Med 2021;27(3):411–8.

65. Lu H, Tan Y, Xie Q. Preliminary observation of deep cervical lymphatic- venous anastomosis using off-eye piece 3d microscope to treat an elderly patient with cognitive impairment. Chinese Journal of Microsurgery 2022;45(5):570–4.

66. Xie Q, Louveau A, Pandey S, et al. Rewiring the Brain – the Next Frontier in Supermicrosurgery. Plast Reconstr Surg 2023. https://doi.org/10.1097/prs. 0000000000010933.

UNITED STATES POSTAL SERVICE® — Statement of Ownership, Management, and Circulation (All Periodicals Publications Except Requester Publications)

1. Publication Title: ORAL & MAXILLOFACIAL SURGERY CLINICS OF NORTH AMERICA

2. Publication Number: 006 – 362

3. Filing Date: 9/18/2024

4. Issue Frequency: FEB, MAY, AUG, NOV

5. Number of Issues Published Annually: 4

6. Annual Subscription Price: $417.00

7. Complete Mailing Address of Known Office of Publication (Not printer) (Street, city, county, state, and ZIP+4®):
ELSEVIER INC.
230 Park Avenue, Suite 800
New York, NY 10169

Contact Person: Malathi Samayan
Telephone (Include area code): 91-44-4299-4507

8. Complete Mailing Address of Headquarters or General Business Office of Publisher (Not printer):
ELSEVIER INC.
230 Park Avenue, Suite 800
New York, NY 10169

9. Full Names and Complete Mailing Addresses of Publisher, Editor, and Managing Editor (Do not leave blank)

Publisher (Name and complete mailing address):
Dolores Meloni, ELSEVIER INC.
1600 JOHN F KENNEDY BLVD. SUITE 1600
PHILADELPHIA, PA 19103-2899

Editor (Name and complete mailing address):
JOHN VASSALLO, ELSEVIER INC.
1600 JOHN F KENNEDY BLVD. SUITE 1600
PHILADELPHIA, PA 19103-2899

Managing Editor (Name and complete mailing address):
PATRICK MANLEY, ELSEVIER INC.
1600 JOHN F KENNEDY BLVD. SUITE 1600
PHILADELPHIA, PA 19103-2899

10. Owner (Do not leave blank. If the publication is owned by a corporation, give the name and address of the corporation immediately followed by the names and addresses of all stockholders owning or holding 1 percent or more of the total amount of stock. If not owned by a corporation, give the names and addresses of the individual owners. If owned by a partnership or other unincorporated firm, give its name and address as well as those of each individual owner. If the publication is published by a nonprofit organization, give its name and address.)

Full Name	Complete Mailing Address
WHOLLY OWNED SUBSIDIARY OF REED/ELSEVIER, US HOLDINGS	1600 JOHN F KENNEDY BLVD. SUITE 1600 PHILADELPHIA, PA 19103-2899

11. Known Bondholders, Mortgagees, and Other Security Holders Owning or Holding 1 Percent or More of Total Amount of Bonds, Mortgages, or Other Securities. If none, check box → ☑ None

Full Name	Complete Mailing Address
N/A	

12. Tax Status (For completion by nonprofit organizations authorized to mail at nonprofit rates) (Check one)
The purpose, function, and nonprofit status of this organization and the exempt status for federal income tax purposes:
☑ Has Not Changed During Preceding 12 Months
☐ Has Changed During Preceding 12 Months (Publisher must submit explanation of change with this statement)

PS Form **3526**, July 2014 [Page 1 of 4 (see instructions page 4)] PSN: 7530-01-000-9931 PRIVACY NOTICE: See our privacy policy on www.usps.com.

---

13. Publication Title: ORAL & MAXILLOFACIAL SURGERY CLINICS OF NORTH AMERICA

14. Issue Date for Circulation Data Below: AUGUST 2024

15. Extent and Nature of Circulation

		Average No. Copies Each Issue During Preceding 12 Months	No. Copies of Single Issue Published Nearest to Filing Date
a. Total Number of Copies (Net press run)		348	329
b. Paid Circulation (By Mail and Outside the Mail)	(1) Mailed Outside-County Paid Subscriptions Stated on PS Form 3541 (Include paid distribution above nominal rate, advertiser's proof copies, and exchange copies)	283	265
	(2) Mailed In-County Paid Subscriptions Stated on PS Form 3541 (Include paid distribution above nominal rate, advertiser's proof copies, and exchange copies)	0	0
	(3) Paid Distribution Outside the Mails Including Sales Through Dealers and Carriers, Street Vendors, Counter Sales, and Other Paid Distribution Outside USPS®	50	49
	(4) Paid Distribution by Other Classes of Mail Through the USPS (e.g., First-Class Mail®)	8	8
c. Total Paid Distribution (Sum of 15b (1), (2), (3) and (4))		341	322
d. Free or Nominal Rate Distribution (By Mail and Outside the Mail)	(1) Free or Nominal Rate Outside-County Copies included on PS Form 3541	6	6
	(2) Free or Nominal Rate In-County Copies Included on PS Form 3541	0	0
	(3) Free or Nominal Rate Copies Mailed at Other Classes Through the USPS (e.g., First-Class Mail)	0	0
	(4) Free or Nominal Rate Distribution Outside the Mail (Carriers or other means)	1	1
e. Total Free or Nominal Rate Distribution (Sum of 15d (1), (2), (3) and (4))		7	7
f. Total Distribution (Sum of 15c and 15e)		348	329
g. Copies not Distributed (See Instructions to Publishers #4 (page #3))		0	0
h. Total (Sum of 15f and g)		348	329
i. Percent Paid (15c divided by 15f times 100)		98.13%	97.87%

* If you are claiming electronic copies, go to line 16 on page 3. If you are not claiming electronic copies, skip to line 17 on page 3.

PS Form **3526**, July 2014 (Page 2 of 4)

16. Electronic Copy Circulation

		Average No. Copies Each Issue During Preceding 12 Months	No. Copies of Single Issue Published Nearest to Filing Date
a. Paid Electronic Copies	▲		
b. Total Paid Print Copies (Line 15c) + Paid Electronic Copies (Line 16a)	▲		
c. Total Print Distribution (Line 15f) + Paid Electronic Copies (Line 16a)	▲		
d. Percent Paid (Both Print & Electronic Copies) (16b divided by 16c × 100)	▲		

☑ I certify that 50% of all my distributed copies (electronic and print) are paid above a nominal price.

17. Publication of Statement of Ownership
☑ If the publication is a general publication, publication of this statement is required. Will be printed in the NOVEMBER 2024 issue of this publication. ☐ Publication not required.

18. Signature and Title of Editor, Publisher, Business Manager, or Owner

Malathi Samayan — Malathi Samayan - Distribution Controller

Date: 9/18/2024

I certify that all information furnished on this form is true and complete. I understand that anyone who furnishes false or misleading information on this form or who omits material or information requested on the form may be subject to criminal sanctions (including fines and imprisonment) and/or civil sanctions (including civil penalties).

PS Form **3526**, July 2014 (Page 3 of 4) PRIVACY NOTICE: See our privacy policy on www.usps.com.

Moving?

Make sure your subscription moves with you!

To notify us of your new address, find your **Clinics Account Number** (located on your mailing label above your name), and contact customer service at:

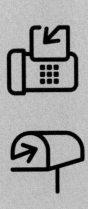

Email: journalscustomerservice-usa@elsevier.com

800-654-2452 (subscribers in the U.S. & Canada)
314-447-8871 (subscribers outside of the U.S. & Canada)

Fax number: 314-447-8029

**Elsevier Health Sciences Division
Subscription Customer Service
3251 Riverport Lane
Maryland Heights, MO 63043**

ELSEVIER